PHOTOGRAPHY
by NAZLI DEVELI

DESIGN
by STUDIO AURORA

EDITOR
STELLA NILSSON

Hardcover Edition - First Printing, February 2022
ISBN 9781736374290
Independently published by Nazlı Develi

www.gurmevegan.com
www.greenandawake.com

GREEN & AWAKE

FOOD WE LOVE

FEEL-GOOD WHOLESOME PLANT-BASED RECIPES FROM SCRATCH

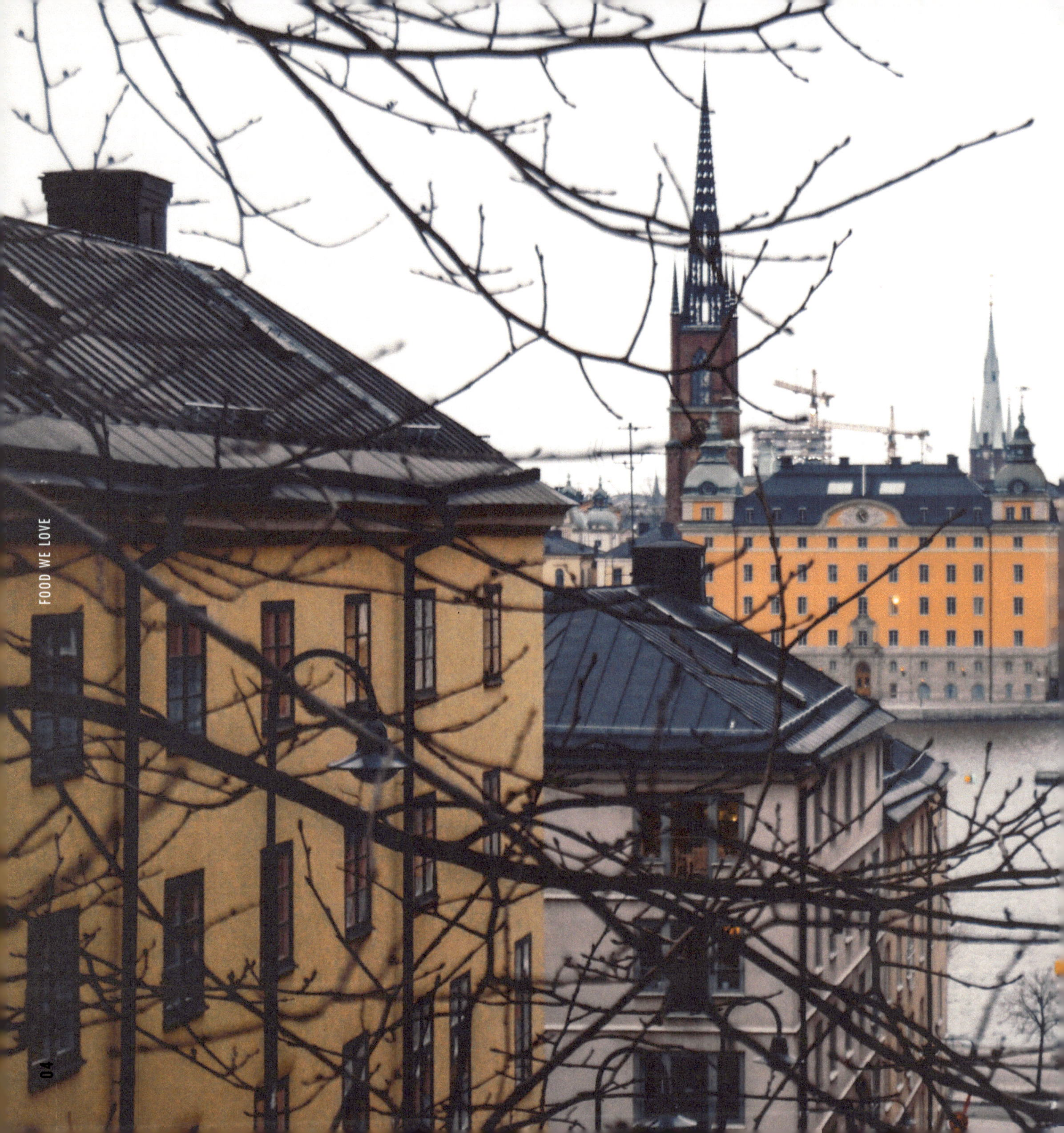

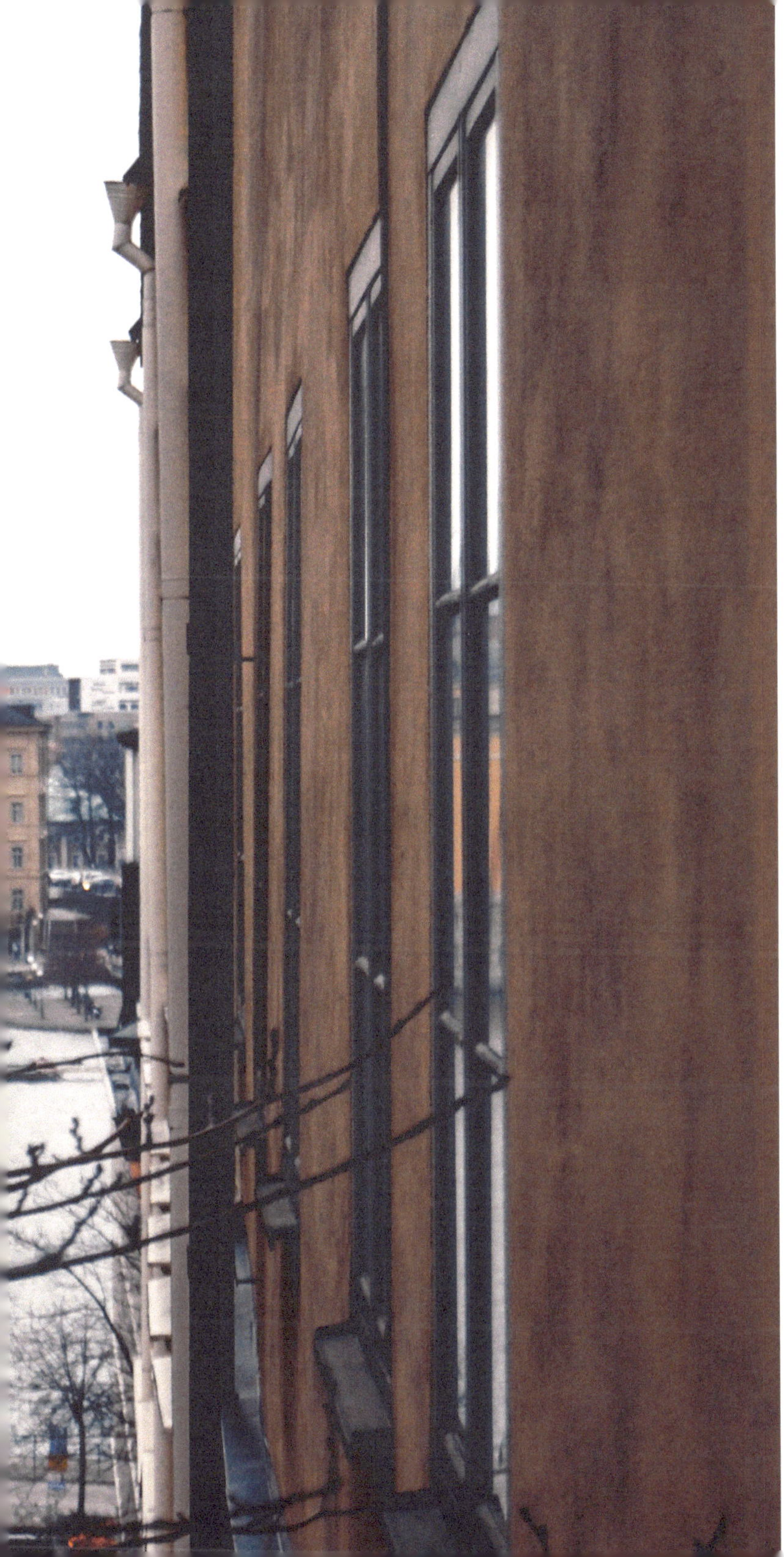

CONTENT

NOTHING TASTES AS GOOD AS HEALTHY FEELS...

INTRODUCTION

"Food We Love" is a new elevated gluten-free and whole food vegan cookbook to celebrate everyday moments with delicious recipes that will bring a little comfort and feeling good vibes to you.
The whole food plant-based diet goes back to the roots of true home cooking by using plants in their natural state. I love clean gourmet food and I believe that gourmet food can be simple yet delicious – in its purest form, as little processed as possible so you can get the most out of it and its true taste is never masked.

My concept is based health values and my food is always made from scratch with organic ingredients, seasonal, local and sustainable as much as possible, never deep fried and processed oil-free and also free from gluten, yeast, dairy and refined sugar.

I am not perfect when it comes to sustainability, it is not easy... But trying to do my best and I truly believe to the saying 'we do not need a handful of people being sustainable perfectly, but millions of people doing it imperfectly.'

Over the years, my primary purpose has been very clear: to develop high-vibrational conscious dining experiences that nourishes the body and soul, awakens all the senses – *not just the taste but attention to detail.*

In this book, you will find almost 100 recipes - packed with the nutrients and taste that nature intended, with high levels of vitamins, minerals, fibre and antioxidants which nourishes our cells, keeps us healthy and feeling good.

I want you to play with the trick that makes vegetables cook cleaner, feel healthier, and taste far more flavorful. Not only just recipes, this cookbook will also help you free yourself from the bonds of recipes with my tips. There are simple ingredient swaps and tips that indicate how you can tweak the recipe to suit your own individual needs. Therefore you can develop your own clean recipes at any time and with the ingredients you have on hand.

Food Designer, Chef & Author

BEFORE YOU GET STARTED

Food We Love ingredients are used in their nature state as much as possible. Below you will find the common ingredients, equipments and cooking methods used in this book.

Sweeteners

The recipes in this book have no refined sugars at all, just use whole foods to sweeten. Because refined sugar is processed, which means the fiber and nutrients are taken out. Without fiber, sugar rushes through our system which causes spikes and dips in blood sugar and increases our risk for developing serious health issues like chronic inflammation, heart disease, type 2 diabetes, and certain types of cancer.

These whole-food sweeteners include: dates, bananas, pumpkins, apples, figs, raisins, apricots, peaches, tamarind and other dried and fresh fruits. It is easy to make your own date puree by blending soaked dates with water until you've reached a smooth consistency. Dates are loaded with both fiber and natural sugar and have a rich, molasses-like taste that will give your dessert a unique flavor. Try making syrup from raisins or different varieties of dates such as sukkari for a caramel-like flavour or acve, figs or prunes for a more distinctive flavor.

You can also use natural less-refined sources of sugar like real maple syrup. Maple is better than refined sugars like granulated sugar and high fructose corn, agave or rice syrup. Agave syrup is marketed with a low glycemic index. But very high in fructose and nobody talks about this. Fructose, in its simplest form, can be processed by the body only from fruits.

If you are looking for an inexpensive alternative to maple, grape molasses without sugar works great. Grapes are reduced by simmering until becomes syrupy. It's a natural sweetener that has been used a lot in ancient times. Make sure to buy a natural one, most of them include sugar addition, or make your own molasses from the sweet fruits grown in your country.

Nuts and Seeds

I usually use walnuts, almonds, hazelnuts, hemp hearts, flaxseeds, chia, black and white sesame, pumpkin seeds and sunflower seeds in my recipes. I do not prefer cashews due to their unethical production conditions today. I also avoid other tropical nuts as much as possible and prefer my local alternatives.

Blender and Food Processor

They are essential to make the smooth and thick mixtures, creams, sauces and soups. For liquid mixtures, a high speed blender works best. Food processors are usually used for dough-like textures and vegetable or fruit chopping. A high speed blender also will help you making seed, nut butters and fruit powders.

Oils and Butters

I avoid all kind of bottled (processed) oils in my recipes. I strongly believe that it is always **the best to have healthy fats in fruit form; from whole nuts, fruits, greens and seeds.** All plant-based foods contain healthy essential fats – just like they have protein and carbohydrates. I use vegetable broth and water for sautéing and frying. In baked goods, nut butters and fruit purées like mashed banana and dates are very good whole food plant-based ingredients we love in our kitchen.

What Led Us To Oil-Free?

First, all the bottled oils are the fatty part of what was a whole food. When we extract the oil, we leave behind the vast majority of these nutrients, and what remains is a very concentrated source of fat and calories without health benefits.

And all the bottled oils such as coconut oil, avocado oil, olive oil, grapeseed oil, almond oil, hemp oil and other seed oils are highly refined. Once oil is extracted from the sources it is considered toxic and it is very high in calories. One tablespoon of olive oil has 120 calories and 14 grams of fat. Coconut oil is also 90% saturated fat.

The next, oil consumption also leads to inflammation in our blood. Many industries have an interest in keeping us eating the highly processed foods they sell.

Oil, even olive oil which is marketed as healthy, inflames the arteries which is the first step in the body sending cholesterol to the inflammation trying to bandage off the inflammation. After years of this irritation, the plaques can either choke off the artery or rupture their pus filled contents into the blood stream which contributes to arterial damage and results to the heart attack.

We do need fat from different sources in our diet but fat from bottled oil is not one of those sources. We do already get these necessary oils from the food we consume daily.

One can eat the seeds, nuts, fruits in small quantity and get the little doses of the fats we need, in low-calorie amounts, and healthy disease preventing packages, that our body recognizes and can use to make us healthy.

The food prepared conventionally is also heavy, greasy and doesn't taste good. The oil literally coats the tongue and blocks the flavor of the food we eat from getting to our taste buds. In the early days, you do yearn for oil, but as time goes on, you will come to appreciate the good taste of the food you now eat without oil and appreciate knowing that this is a wonderfully healthy way to feed your body. Cooking without oils can be a bit challenging for beginners, but it certainly can be done easily. The studies concluded that, on average, it takes 66 days for a new behavior to become automatic. You just have to find ways to replace the moisture and other properties the oil imparts.

Oil also masks flavor. With dry roasting, each vegetable's subtlety comes through in entirely different ways. Summer squash gets this incredible tropical aroma, like really ripe mango or papaya but more vegetal.

We all know water and oil don't mix as the oil molecule is non polar. Its charge is evenly balanced rather than having one positive and one negative end. This means oil molecules are more attracted to other oil molecules than water molecules, and water molecules are more attracted to each other than oil, so the two never mix. So when vegetables cooked in oil, eventually the water content hits a steaming point. It reacts with the oil. It splatters. It makes the kitchen stink. It's a mess to clean up. Our preference to dry roast—to cook vegetables entirely naked and then immediately seasonings afterward.

There are some special tips when roasting without oil, and I have covered the ways in this book.

However, if you absolutely prefer to use some oil, it would be better to add a high quality extra virgin olive oil or nut oil, just add after you have finished the cooking process, because oil becomes much more toxic when heated.

Choosing The Correct Baking Pan

It is very important to choose the right cookware while you are cooking without oil in order to prevent sticking. Some good options are heavy-bottomed stainless steel pans, enamel-coated cast iron, or ceramic titanium pans. Silicone ovenware is great for easy release when baking oil-free sweets. Parchment paper is also a wonderful option to line baking sheets and casserole dishes.

For a successful in oil-free cooking please also remember that the pan needs to be big enough. Just large enough so the veggies can have a breathing room. Never smoosh them together so tightly in a dish that the heat won't be able to get at all sides of the veggie properly or they won't cook evenly.

Avocados and Nut Butters

In desserts, I usually use seed butters or nut butters. To make your own nut or seed butter, simply place the nuts/seeds into a high speed blender and process for couple of minutes until you get creamy butter. You can roast them before making butter, this makes the process easier or use as raw.

I also love to use whole avocado - the healthiest fat in the world. Avocado was known as a butter fruit in ancient times and was used a lot. However, we recommend its consumption in fruit form, not in bottled oil form.

I try to avoid the use of coconut as much as much as possible as it is not local and in order to avoid cruelty , but I agree that coconut butter works well in certain recipes. (It is not an issue for those who are living in the tropics, sure.) I try to prefer local products as much as possible, when needed to use imported one, pay attention to fair trade label, choose the companies who do not use monkeys or human children to harvest coconuts. I believe this is our responsibility for the future of world.

What About Salt?

Recipes in this book use pink himalayan salt or flaked sea salt. But I use very small amount of salt and mostly blend the salt with salt alternatives to minimalize the amount of the salt.
If you're having trouble eating without salt / or less salt, oil, and sugar but wanting to go this way, doing a weekly juice detox can help restore your palate.

It is said that sodium controls fluid balance in our bodies and maintains blood volume and blood pressure. Eating too much sodium may raise blood pressure and cause fluid retention, which could lead to swelling of the legs and feet or other health issues.

Up to half of our salt intake is from processed food, with the balance occurring naturally in food and water. Foods that contain significant amounts of potassium and also low levels of sodium are fresh fruits and vegetables.
Common salt alternatives you may want to use are celery powder, celery juice, peppercorns, fresh lemon juice with the dulse, wakame, nori blend and other seaweed varieties.

This book is not a prescription and there is no one right way that works for everyone. I believe the necessity of a good balance. When we use something a lot and regularly and turn this into a habit, we may feel the harmful effects in the long term. Instead of cutting the salt completely it is best to use a pinch. A pinch of salt also adds dimension to the desserts.

Plant-based Milks

Recipes in this book usually use oat or almond milk. These two make an easy match without changing the taste of the recipe. You can also use hazelnut or walnut for a more nutty taste, or coconut milk for a sweeter taste if you prefer.
You can get store-bought or make your own milk at home. But the best way is to make yourself. Only three almonds are enough for 500 ml water. After blending them, strain through a cheesecloth. Remove the pulp to use later (you can dehydrate then process into flour), use the strained milk in your recipes.

Flours

I use buckwheat and oat flour a lot. For optimal digestion, soak the buckwheats/whole oats in the water to activate, then allow to sprout, dehydrate and blend into fine flour or use packaged sprouted buckwheat/oat flour if you find this easier. Both regular buckwheat flour and sprouted one work well in the recipes. For the oat flour, you can simply blend the gluten-free rolled oats in a high speed blender (I use Blendtec, it works great to make fine flour and silky smooth creams. It is really worth to invest to a good blender) until you get fine flour.

Binders and Thickeners

Cassava, tapioca, arrowroot, taro, sprouted brown rice flour, chia seeds, flaxseeds and psyllium husk powder are the some ingredients I use as a binder and thickener in the recipes.

Cassava flour is a great gluten-free substitute for tapioca flour. Arrowroot contains more fiber, making it a more nutrient-dense option. Tapioca and cassava are made from cassava root, but cassava flour incorporates the whole root, whereas tapioca flour is made up of only the starchy part of the plant.

Tapioca is a starch extracted from the cassava root through a process of washing and pulping. The wet pulp is then squeezed to extract a starchy liquid. Once all the water evaporates from the starchy liquid, the tapioca flour remains. So it is refined one. Arrowroot starch is also similar to tapioca's process. It is extracted from the root of plant.

The whole food logic is simple, part of a vegetable should not be extracted, but the whole should be used. A portion of which starch is extracted, oil is squeezed and sugar is taken should not be used.

If the plant is dried and turned into flour, it is partially more acceptable because it partially contains starch, sugar and oil.

The cassava flour is the whole root, simply peeled, dried and ground. This makes it best ingredient as a thickener.

These were some of my gluten-free preferences. But I am pretty aware of there is no one clear right way to do things. The right way varies from person to person and depending on situations. So feel free to play with the ingredients and choose whatever best suits to you. If you can't find cassava, you can use tapioca or arrowroot of course as sometimes I did. I don't prefer potato, white rice or corn starch. It if suits to you, you can use them where I used cassava or tapioca in this book.

Taro is also wonderful strachy root vegetable, similar to potato. You can dehydrate and grind it into flour to use as a binder in the gluten-free flour mixtures.

Why We Don't Use Nutritional Yeast Anymore?

Not only nutritional yeast, actually I don't use any kind of yeast.
Nutritional yeast is produced by culturing a yeast in a nutrient medium for several days. The primary ingredient in the growth medium is glucose, often from either sugarcane or beet molasses. When the yeast is ready, it is deactivated with heat and then harvested, washed, dried and packaged. It contains naturally occurring MSG. Monosodium glutamate works slowly and insidiously on the human brain, and it is hard to measure its effects on those who don't have a glutamate sensitivity. While nutritional yeast contains amino acids, minerals, and B vitamins, there are better food sources for this nutrition that are not man-made. Whole food logic simple: eating plants in their natural state is the best.

Why We don't Use Aquafaba?

Aquafaba - chickpea water, in particular, is useful for whipping up egg-free desserts.
Since aquafaba was found, it has become very popular. But I haven't heard about people that would voluntarily drink water from cooked legumes. The soaking and boiling water is normally unwanted thing, a waste. The soaking water is poured off, when chickpeas are cooked. And we remove their skins. As the legumes cook, all foam that rises to the top of the cooking water is carefully skimmed off. Sometimes water is replaced midway during the cooking process. Such care in preparation ensures that legumes will be thoroughly digestible. This indicates they were attempting to get rid of something. In raw cuisine, we also soak legumes and remove the water, rinse many times then leave to sprout them. When we sprout them, we get rid of phytic acid, and they become more digestible. Whenever I create a recipe, I design it to be as health-building as possible. Knowing where it comes from - the slimy brine - doesn't entince us in the slightest. There are far too many elements of aquafaba that are detrimental to our health for it to be somethig we would use. For instance; saponins, oligosaccharides, phytic acid. Saponins are a toxic steroid derivative that disrupts red blood cells. They also contribute to the development of leaky gut over time by damaging the gut wall. Saponins are thermally sensitive and dissolve in water when soaked or blanched causing a detergent-like effect. If you are not aware of this, please observe the water when you cook chickpeas, beans or grains in your pot next time. You will notice the bubbles.
Aquafaba contains a compound known as oligosaccharides. This means that there are sugars in the food that your body can't digest until they reach your colon. The result is bloating and gas, symptoms many people aren't fond of.

Personally I would rather have a flatter cake or non-airy mousse than incorporate aquafaba.
If you have no issue with the aquafaba, you can absolutely use it. But as we don't prefer, there is no aquafaba recipes in this book.

Umami

I don't like common man-made processed umami shortcuts such as soy sauce, miso, yeast, pickles and other fermented stuff. We can get umami flour from the plants with slow cooking methods and right food combinations. For example, we enchance the depth of flavour of the tomatoes with some seaweed varieties naturally by slowly cooking method and dried mushroom water, mushroom powders are great options for natural umami flavour. Some recipes in this book call mushroom stock (page 30) or vegetable jus (page 31), if you prefer you can use tamari or coconut aminos as a gluten-free alternative in the place of them.

Time

All recipes in this book have rough time estimates. Because the actual time varies from person to person depending on your experience and the equipments you have.
But I do believe the estimate time will give you an indication of whether it takes too long or short.

Measurements

A digital kitchen scale is a must when baking gluten-free. Weighing will give you consistent results every time. When you weighed 1 cup buckwheat flour using different volume measuring cups, as a test, you will notice every singe one gives a different amount of grams.
I developed my recipes using grams and converted small amounts to a volume measure to stay as standart as possible. But the best way is to use scale if you can.

The Taste

Vegetables vary in size, variety, flavour, texture depending on season, ripeness, where and in which soil they have been growing.
Even I have covered my recipes detailed in the instructions parts, they may not have the same dish taste in your kitchen. I tried to make the recipes easy and instructive as much as possible, but I kindly do ask that you taste dishes before you serve them, season according to your taste, check the texture, thickness and creamness.

SAUCES ARE THE TRUE TREASURES. YOU CAN MASTER ANY DISH IF YOU KNOW THESE TREASURES WELL ENOUGH.

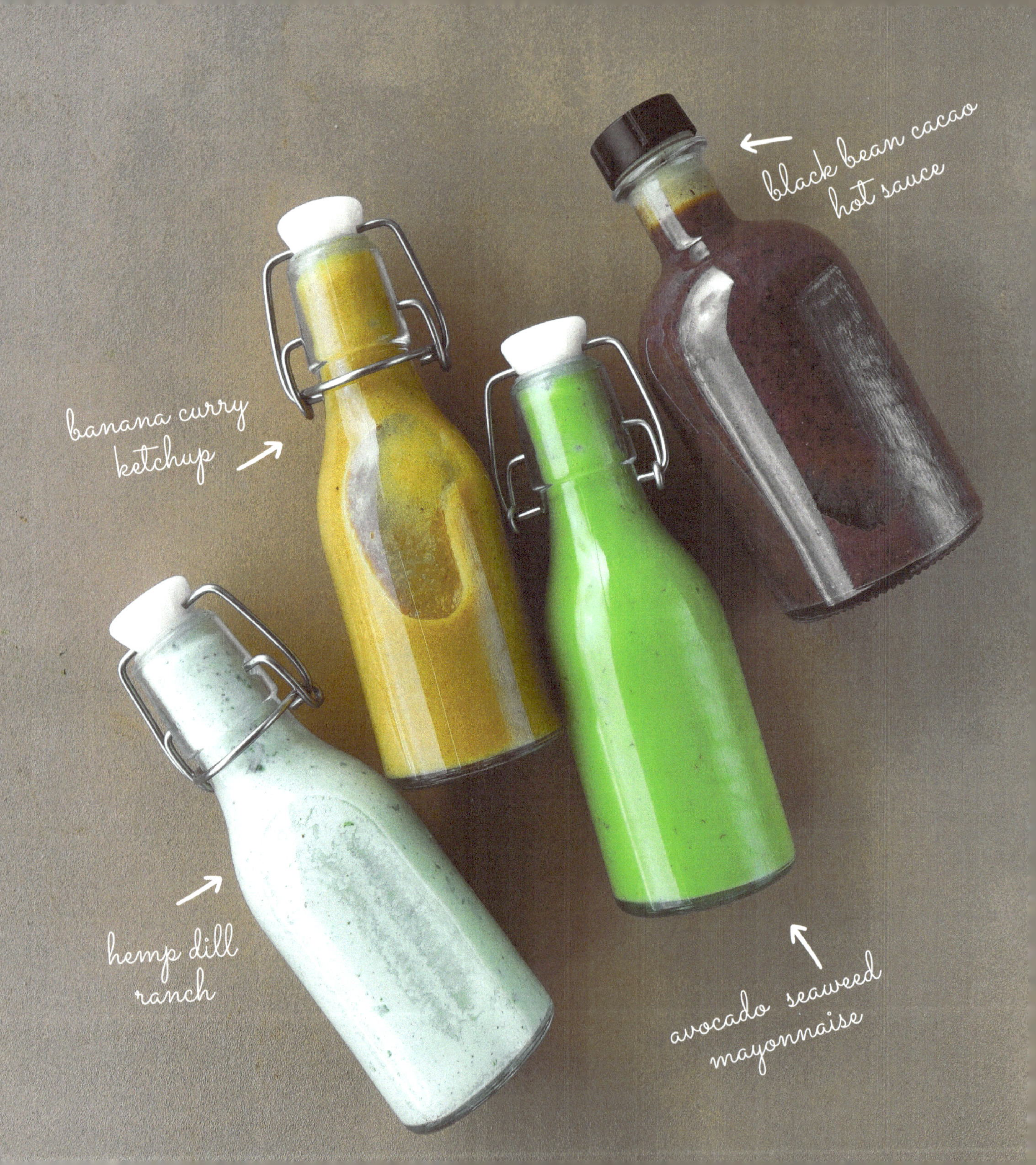
black bean cacao hot sauce
banana curry ketchup
hemp dill ranch
avocado seaweed mayonnaise

HEALTHY CONDIMENTS FROM SCRATCH

Whether it's a party time or just dinner for one, there's always something that doesn't quite make it on the grocery list. That's particularly true for condiments. Making your own condiments is healthier and definitely less wasteful.

Makes 1 small 220 ml bottle of each

Avocado Seaweed Mayonnaise

1 ripe avocado
150 ml filtered water
5 tbsp lemon juice
1 tsp ground mustard
1/2 shallot chopped finely
1 tsp dulse powder
2 garlic cloves minced
1/4 tsp salt

Peel your avocado, remove the seed. Place in a high speed blender.
Add the lemon juice, mustard, shallot, garlic, filtered water, dulse and salt.
Blend until silky smooth.
Pour in the glass bottles. Keep in the refrigerator up to 3 days.

TIPS - Use any kind of seaweed such as dulse, nori, wakame in fine powder form.

Banana Curry Ketchup

1 small yellow onion
2 garlic cloves
1 tsp curry powder
4 tbsp beetroot broth (page 25)
175 g bananas
50 ml water
50 ml lime juice
2 large medjool dates pitted
1/2 tsp salt

Peel and chop the onion and garlic.
Cook in 2 tablespoons of beet water for about 3 minutes. Then add the curry powder and whisk.
Then add the bananas. Pour over water and lime juice. Mix in the dates. Let simmer without lid for about 20 min.
Mix the ketchup smoothly with the rest of 2 tablespoons beet broth. Season with salt. Let cool. Pour in to the glass jar. Keep in the refrigerator.

TIPS - You can also use fresh peach, apricot or mango in the place of banana.

Hemp Seed Ranch

75 g hemp hearts (a.k.a hulled hemp seeds)
1/4 bunch fresh dill chopped
1 spring green onion chopped
1 tsp dijon mustard
Juice of whole lemon
1 garlic clove minced
1/4 medium white onion
60 ml plant milk (hemp, oat or almond)
A pinch of sea and ground black pepper

Place all ingredients in a high speed blender. Blend until smooth.
Pour in to the glass jars. Refrigerate for 2 hours before using.

TIPS - Hemp heart replacments can be sunflower seeds, pine nuts, almonds, fair trade cashews or macadamia nuts.

Black Bean Cacao Hot Sauce

60 g black beans cooked
1 yellow onion chopped
2 garlic cloves minced
1 jalapeño chopped
1/4 cup (60 ml) beet broth for cooking + 3-4 tbsp to thin as needed
1 tbsp espresso cold
2 tbsp mushroom stock (page 30)
1 tsp maple syrup
1 tsp cacao (or carob)
200 ml water
1 tsp white wine vinegar
1/4 tsp salt

Put the beans in cold water for about 12 hours or over-night. Then cook until soften.
Peel and chop the onion and garlic. Fry onion, garlic and jalapeño in 1/4 cup beet broth on high heat so it turns really brown.
Add the cacao (or carob), mushroom stock (or tamari), maple and coffee. Stir well. Let the beans drain and mix them into the mixture. Add the 200 ml water. Cook together until everything combined well and thick. Taste with vinegar and season with salt. Add 3-4 tbsp beet broth to thin the mixture.
Transfer mixture in a high speed blender, blend until smooth.
Transfer back to the pot, heat on medium heat by con-stanly stirring for about 1-2 minutes.

HOW TO USE? - Serve with your sandwich, wrap or bowl. It is also great to brush vegetable balls.

Fresh Tomato Ketchup

3 cups chopped tomatoes
1/2 cup red onion finely chopped
1 cup beet juice freshly juiced
6-7 medjool dates pitted and chopped
1/4 cup lemon juice
1 tsp chili powder
1/4 tsp freshly ground black pepper
1/4 cup no salt added tomato paste
1/2 tsp salt

In a pot on medium heat, combined the tomatoes, onions, beet juice and chopped dates.
Bring to boiling over medium; reduce heat. Simmer, uncovered, about 30 minutes or until vegetables are tender. Remove from heat; let cool slightly.
Transfer tomato mixture to a blender. Add the remaining ingredients and 1 cup water. Cover and blend until smooth. Clean saucepan and return mixture to pan. Bring to boiling; reduce heat to medium. Simmer 1 to 1½ hours or until mixture reduces to a thick paste, stirring frequently.
Meanwhile, prepare the sauce bottles with caps. Bring a large pot of water to boiling. Submerge bottles and lids in the water; boil for 10 minutes. Use tongs to remove jars and lids from water and drain; transfer to a cooling rack or towel.
Working quickly, pour the hot ketchup into the sterilized bottles and close tightly. Cool completely.

Keep in the refrigerator. In unopened sterilized jars or bottles, ketchup will keep 6 months. Once opened, ketchup keeps up to 1 month.

Barbecue Sauce

400 g homemade tomato sauce
1 tsp chili pepper
1/2 tsp mustard powder
1 tsp garlic powder (or asafoetida)
1 tbsp apple cider vinegar
1 tbsp maple syrup
1 small shallot peeled and grated (or asafoetida)
2 tbsp intense mushroom stock (or 1 tbsp tamari or coconut aminos)
1/4 tsp black pepper and salt to taste

Place all ingredients in a blender, blend until smooth. Pour mixture in a small saucepan, let it cook for 10 minutes on medium heat until thicken.
Transfer mixture in a glass jar. Store in the refrigerator.

Asafoetida - As an onion & garlic replacement

Asafoetida is a gum from a variety of giant fennel, which naturally has a strong and pungent smell, rather like rotting garlic (as in foetid). It's a very useful spice for those who can't or won't eat onion or garlic, as it adds a similar depth and savouriness to food. It can help with the symptoms of irritable bowel syndrome.

You can replace onion and garlic with the asafoetida powder. Small amounts of asafoetida give a comforting onion-garlic flavour. 1/2 teaspoon of the powder can be substituted for 2 minced garlic cloves or 2/3 of a cup of minced onion.

You will find asafoetida in its powdered form at Indian, Middle Eastern and Asian markets. It usually has two forms. First, it comes as a brown powder. This type is known as the full-strength version and is extremely powerful in terms of smell. I highly advise you to use very small pinches of this version when you cook with it.
Second, you can source asafoetida as a yellow powder. This version generally involves turmeric and/or rice powder. It is much milder, so perhaps try this one first.

TOPPINGS

Below you will find my favorite toppings. They are very versatile and will rock any kind of dish, can be made beforehand and stored up to 2-3 months in the airtight container.

Chickpea Crumb

200 g roasted chickpeas
75 g toasted pine nuts (or walnuts)
1/2 tsp garlic powder
1/2 tsp lemon peel powder or lemon zest
1/2 tsp salt
1/4 tsp chili pepper

In a food processor, combine the roasted chickpeas and pine nuts or walnuts, garlic powder, lemon zest, and salt to taste. Pulse until you have a crumbly mixture.
Store in the glass jar up to 2-3 months.

Celeriac Crumb

1 large head celeriac
2 tbsp mushroom stock (page 30)
1 tsp dulse powder
Salt and pepper to taste
1 tbsp toasted sesame seeds
3 tbsp gluten-free breadcrumbs (page 158)

Peel the celeriac. Transfer to a food processor, blend until rice-like texture. Then add the mushroom stock, dulse, salt and pepper. Massage well. Transfer mixture on a parchment paper. Spread as thin as possible. Bake in the oven at 170° C with fan until completely dried and crispy. Then mix with the toasted sesame seeds and gluten-free breadcrumbs. Store in the airtight container. It also can be used as it is, without sesame and breadcrumbs. Add to your salad, pasta or risotto dishes to enchance to flavour and texture. You can also make mushroom version of this crumb by adding 400 g diced mushrooms + 1 tbsp tomato paste and +1 tsp dulse to the same recipe.

Sunflower Hemp Crumb

130 g sunflower seeds
40 g hemp hearts
1 tsp garlic powder
1 tsp dried lemon zest
1/2 tsp onion powder (or asafoetida, page 22)
1/2 tsp salt

Mix everything in a high speed blender, transfer to a glass jar. When a recipe call nut parmesan in this book, I use this recipe. You can make your own or use your favorite plant-based parmesan.

Store in the glass jar up to 2-3 months.

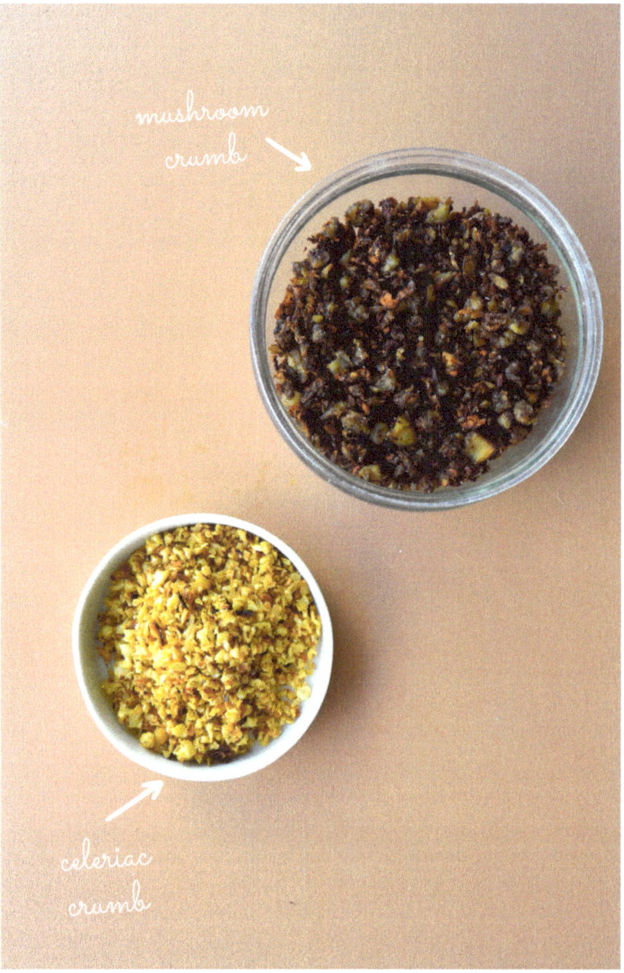
mushroom
crumb
celeriac
crumb

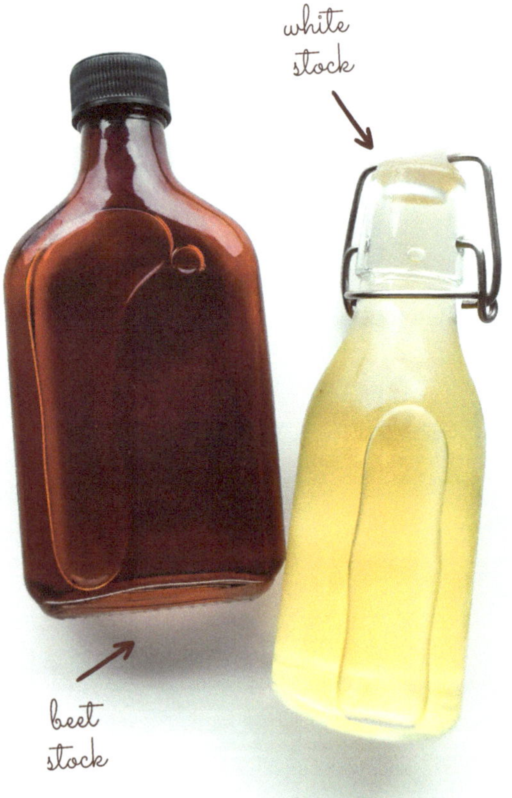
white
stock
beet
stock

VEGETABLE STOCKS

Vegetable stocks are used as the essential of many dishes to improve their depth of flavour. They are healthier, when no fat is used to cook the vegetables.

The stock can be made from ends, tops and trimmings of the vegetables or from the whole vegetables depending on your choice. For zero waste stocks, it is best to use the vegetables from the leftovers.

There are two basic types of vegetable stock; white and brown.

White vegetable stocks are typically colourless and milder and fresher in taste, adding a subtle flavour to dishes. These are made by simply adding the vegetables raw into a pot with water and simmering.

Brown vegetable stocks are richer and deeper in colour, adding a more robust flavour to dishes. This is achieved by roasting the vegetables until caramelised, before simmering them in water.

WHICH VEGETABLES WORK BEST?

For a base, start with onion, garlic, celery, leek, cauliflower, carrot and peppers. The standard aromatics are bay leaves, peppercorns, thyme, rosemary, dill and parsley stalks. You can then add other vegetables, herbs or spices to flavour your stock however you want.

Use sunchokes or celeriac for an earthier taste, butternut squash peel or apple for sweeter notes or fennel, star anise, cardamom and some tarragon for a stock with a pleasant aniseed flavour.

For a light stock, use a white stock base and add pea pods, kohlrabi, artichoke leaves, woody asparagus ends or bean pods.

Use beetroot stock from the cooked beetroots for a versatile stock. It works wonderful to saute the onions and garlic. You will find so many recipes that call beetroot broth in this book. It is my absolute favorite I've found by experimenting recently. To make, simply wash 2-3 medium beets, place in a pot. Cover with water and boil until soften. Strain and collect the water from the beets. Store in the glass bottle in the refrigerator.

vegetable stocks continued

Ginger, tangerine and lemon grass in white stock give you a nice aromatic flavour.

For an intense stock, use the beetroot stock base and add umami-rich ingredients such as dried mushrooms, tomatoes, carrots and seaweeds.

PREPARING THE VEGETABLES

The fresher the vegetables you add for stock, the better the flavour will be. Collect peels, ends and trimmings to add to the pot for extra flavour while cooking and set aside to use in veg stock. It is also important to ensure they have been cleaned well.

All the vegetables should be chopped very finely. This is important because more of the vegetable will be exposed to water while simmering and also creates a larger surface area for caramelisation in the oven.

As a rule, always add an equal amount of water to the weight of the vegetables, or pour water into the pan until the vegetables are fully submerged but covered by no more than a few centimetres.

HOW TO MAKE?

In a large pot, add the vegetables of your preference and sweat down until just starting to colour – around 10 minutes.

If using balsamic, add now and reduce by half. Then top up with water until the vegetables are just covered by a few centimetres. Bring to the boil.

Turn down to a simmer then add the spices such as bay leaves, rosemary, peppercorns or aromatics such as ginger or lemongrass. Continue cooking for at least 30 minutes, preferably 45 minutes to 1 hour. The flavor will deepen the longer it cooks.

Strain through or a strainer so you are left with a nice clear stock. Divide between storage vessels. Let cool completely before sealing. Use immediately or chill it.

The stock will keep for 3–5 days in the fridge or will freeze for up to 2 months

MUSHROOM CAULIFLOWER WHITE STOCK

1 cup cauliflower stems and leaves
1 cup button mushrooms
1 large onion
1/4 cup celery sticks
4 garlic cloves
1 tsp salt
1 bay leaf
1 tbsp mustard seeds
1 tbsp peppercorns
2 lt water

Instructions

Preheat oven to 200° C.
Line a baking tray with parchment paper.
Place the sliced mushrooms, cauliflower stems and leaves, onion and garlic cloves on the parchment.
Roast for 15 minutes or until nicely caramelized. This process will give more flavour to the stock.
Then transfer them in a pot, add the sliced celery, bay leaf, mustard seeds, peppercorns and water. Bring to boil on low-medium heat for 30 minutes.
Once done, strain the stock through a large sieve.

Can be stored in an airtight container in the fridge up to 4 days.

VEGETABLE PEELINGS - VEG STOCK POWDER

This is an easy recipe to make your own vegetable stock powder using peelings and any veg and herbs that need using up. It's really adaptable - feel free to mix it up and experiment each time with whatever peelings, vegetables and herbs you have available. Collect veg peelings in a bag in your freezer for a good few weeks so you have enough to make a bigger batch of stock that will last longer.

Vegetables that work well include onions, garlic, carrots, celery, leeks, parsnip, potato, swede, tomato, broccoli, cauliflower, fennel, kale, mushrooms. You can include herbs too, try parsley, dill, rosemary, thyme, oregano, sage, basil and chives.

Ingredients

Vegetables and/or veg peelings
Fresh herbs of your choice
Sea salt

Instructions

Wash and dry your selection of vegetables, peelings and herbs.
Roughly chop them all, then transfer to a food processor and blend until you've got a very finely chopped consistency, almost like a paste.

You may need to do this stage in batches if you're making a large amount.
Tip the vegetable mix into a large bowl and weigh it. Next, add 20% of the weight in salt, i.e for 200g of veg, add 20g salt. This may seem like a lot, but you will only be adding half teaspoon or so to each meal, and it works as a natural preservative. Mix thoroughly.

Add the salt and vegetable mix to a large saucepan and cook slowly on a low heat for 1-2 hours, stirring occasionally, until the veg is soft and cooked through. If a lot of moisture comes out from the veg during the cooking process, wait until it is all absorbed and cooked off.

vegetable peelings and veg stock powders continued

Line a baking tray with greaseproof paper. Spoon the mixture onto the paper and spread it out evenly. Leave in a dehydrator overnight or slowly dry it out in the oven at 150° C for 1-2 hours, stirring occasionally, until it's completely dry and crisp.
Allow to cool completely, then transfer to your food processor and blend again until you have a fine powder. Store your stock powder in a clean, airtight jar for up to 3 months. Use 1-2 teaspoons to 1 litre of boiling water for a flavourful stock.

MUSHROOM STOCK

1 onion chopped
2 tsp tomato puree/paste
200 g mushrooms roughly chopped (I used shiitake, button or cremini)
15 g dried mushroom powder (shiitake, button or cremini)
3 garlic cloves smashed
2 bay leaves
3 tbsp beetroot stock (page 25)
1 tsp salt
3 black peppercorns
1 lt water

Heat the beet stock in a large pot, then add the carrots and onion. Cook over a high heat until it begins to brown, about 5-6 minutes. Ensure that it browns a bit, as you don't want to sweat the vegetables or the stock will be too sweet. Also, don't get it too dark or it will have a bitter taste.

Stir in the tomato puree/paste and cook for 2 minutes to caramelise. Stir in all the remaining ingredients and bring to the boil, then reduce the heat and simmer for 25-30 minutes.
Place a fine mesh sieve over a large bowl and strain the mushroom stock into it. Discard the solids from the sieve. Then add your mushroom stock back to the pan and simmer for a further 15 minutes to concentrate the flavors. Use immediately or cool and refrigerate for up to 5 days or freeze for up to 3 months.

VEGETABLE JUS

Au jus is a French culinary term meaning "with juice". It refers to dishes prepared or served together with a light broth or gravy. Au jus is a wonderful natural way to enhance the flavour of dishes. You can use this sauce with vegetable steaks like kohlrabi, cauliflower, celeriac or with mashed potatoes, rice, noodles or how you like. This sauce is actually fits all, very versaitle and full of umami.

150 g onion finely chopped
300 g eggplants thinly sliced
100 g carrot thinly sliced
50 g beetroot thinly sliced
100 g broccoli thinly sliced
250 g cauliflower thinly sliced
1 tbsp tomato puree
50 g sliced shitake or porcini
1 tsp salt 4g
10 g seaweed blend (nori,wakame,-dulse)
1 lt filtered water
500 ml beetroot broth
2 g psyllium husk powder

Combine the vegetables with the shitake mushrooms, seaweed, tomato puree and beetroot broth.

Spread evenly on 2 trays and roast in an oven, at 150° C, for 45 minutes.
Scrape roasted vegetables into a stockpot, add the water, and simmer for 40 minutes.

Pass through a chinois, into a clean pot, and reduce by three-quarters.
Whisk in the salt and psyllium.

Best when served immediately but also can be stored. Cool and refrigerate up to 4-5 days. Heat and whisk well before using.

DIPS, SPREADS & SAUCES

BLACK GARLIC TURMERIC HUMMUS

400 g chickpeas cooked
1/2 tsp baking soda
75 g tahini
55 ml lemon juice
1 tsp black garlic puree
1/2 tsp sea salt
1 tsp turmeric powder
3-4 tbsp ice water

Place the pre-cooked chickpeas in a medium saucepan and add the baking soda. Cover the chickpeas with the water, then bring the mixture to a boil over high heat. Continue boiling, reducing heat if necessary to prevent overflow, for about 20 minutes, or until the chickpeas look bloated, their skins are falling off, and they're quite soft. In a fine-mesh strainer, drain the chickpeas and run cool water over them for about 30 seconds. Remove the skins. Strain and set aside.

In a food processor or high-powered blender, combine the lemon juice, black garlic and salt. Process until smooth.
Add the tahini to the food processor and blend until the mixture is thick and creamy, stopping to scrape down any tahini stuck to the sides and bottom of the processor.

While running the food processor, drizzle in 2 tablespoons ice water. Scrape down the food processor, and blend until the mixture is ultra smooth, pale and creamy. (If your tahini was extra-thick to begin with, you might need to add 1 to 2 tablespoons more ice water.)
Add the turmeric and the drained chickpeas to the food processor. Blend until the mixture is super smooth. Add more ice water if necessary to achieve a creamy texture.

Keep in the refrigerator up to 5 days.

AVOCADO GARLIC YOGURT

2 ripe avocados
4-5 tbsp lemon juice
1 garlic clove minced
1/2 tsp salt

Peel and remove the seed your avocado. Place in a blender. Add the rest of the ingredients. Blend until smooth. Add more lemon juice if you like depending on how tangy like and the consistency. The avocados should be very ripe for the best taste.
Keep in the refrigerator up to 3 days.

BEET JEWEL PESTO

100 g cooked beetroots
1.5 tbsp balsamic vinegar or apple juice
1 small red onion chopped
1 garlic cloves minced
2 tbsp pine nuts (or walnuts).
1/4 tsp salt

Cook your beetroots until fork tender. Place in a food processor, process until you get rice-like texture. Add the balsamic, chopped red onion, pine nuts, garlic and salt. Blend to combine everything together. Once done, transfer in a bowl. Serve with your lentil crackers or top on your bread, spread on the sandwich.
Keep in the refrigerator up to 3 days.

BUTTER BEAN WITH TARRAGON DIP

250 g cooked white beans
2 tbsp tahini
50 ml water
Juice of whole lemon
1 tsp salt
A small handful of fresh tarragon
1/4 tsp freshly ground black pepper

Place all the ingredients in a high speed blender, process until you get a smooth creamy texture.
Pour mixture in a glass jar.

It can be stored up to 4 days in the refrigerator.

GREEN OLIVE TAPENADE

150 g green olives
1/4 bunch chopped parsley
1/2 lemon juice
4 tbsp tomato juice
A pinch of salt
1 garlic clove
Fresh tomatoes to top (optional)
4 slices of buckwheat bread

Preheat your oven to 220° C.
Peel the garlic clove and cut it in half. Rub the cut side on both sides of each slice of buckwheat bread to flavour it. Toast in the preheated oven for 5-6 minutes or until crunchy and golden.
In the meantime add all the tapenade ingredients to the small bowl of a food processor with an s-blade. Pulse until you reach the consistency you like. I like mine a little chunky.
Serve while the bread is warm spreading the tapenade onto it and topping with chopped tomatoes if desired.

DANDELION PESTO

90 g fresh dandelion leaves
60 g sunflower seeds or pine nuts
Juice of whole lemon
1/2 tsp salt
1/4 tsp freshly ground black pepper
1 small garlic clove

Place all the ingredients in a high speed blender (like Blendtec with the twister jar), process until you get a smooth puree. Transfer mixture in a glass jar.

Keep in the refrigerator up to 3 days.

RED BELL PEPPER BASIL SPREAD

4 large red bell peppers
80 g sunflower seeds
3 tbsp lemon juice
1/4 tsp pinch of salt
A pinch of cayenne
4-5 fresh basil leaves

Preheat the oven to 200° C. Cut the peppers in half, scoop out the seeds and place on a baking tray. Roast for 30-35 minutes until slightly charred. Once roasted, remove from the oven and leave to cool. Then peel the skin from the peppers, chop and put in a blender. Add the sunflower seeds, cayenne and salt to a skillet and toast for a few minutes on medium heat. Transfer the sunflower seeds,lemon juice and basil leaves and purée until smooth. Put in a glass jar.
Keep in the refrigerator up to 4-5 days.

KIWI AND JALAPENO SALSA VERDE

6 not overly ripe kiwi, peeled and quartered
3 spring onions finely sliced
1 fresh jalapeño deseeded and chopped
1/4 bunch fresh cilantro chopped
Juice of 1 whole lemon
1/2 tsp salt

Place all ingredients in a bowl, mix together. Add the lemon juice and salt. Give it a good toss. Serve with your crispbread.
Keep in the refrigerator up to 2 days.

PICADA SAUCE

2 red bell peppers
4 garlic cloves minced
30 g toasted almonds
30 g toasted pine nuts
1 tsp paprika
Juice of 1 lemon
1/2 bunch parsley chopped

Put the red bell peppers under the grill, turning them occasionally so you blacken each side. Once done, transfer to a bowl, cover with cling-film and allow to cool. Once cool, remove the blackened skins with your hands, then pull the peppers apart and remove the seeds and the stalk.
Add all the ingredients to a food processor, apart from the lemon juice and parsley. Blitz until roughly chopped, then add the lemon juice a little at a time until the consistency is smooth. Transfer to a bowl. Chop the parsley and stir it through, then add the rest of the lemon juice and season with salt and pepper. If you want a slightly crunchier texture, then reserve some of the nuts and add them at the end.

SATAY SAUCE

200 ml peanut butter
100 ml mushroom stock (or coconut aminos, tamari)
20 g lime juice
3 tbsp maple syrup or 4 dates pitted pureed
150 ml oat milk
1 tsp red chili flakes
1 tsp grated fresh ginger
1 garlic clove minced

This indonesian inspired versatile sauce is perfect with salads, broccoli, tempeh, noodles, beans, kale and other greens.

To make, place all ingredients in a blender, blend until smooth. Serve cold with dragon bowl or slightly heat up in a saucepan and serve warm.

Can be stored in an airtight container in the fridge for 3-4 days.

GINGERLY TOMATO SAUCE

1 small red onion
2 tsp minced peeled fresh ginger
2 cloves garlic minced
1/4 cup beetroot broth
2 cups fresh ripe tomatoes peeled diced (if necessary, you may use an equivalent amount of canned tomatoes)
1/2 tsp maple
1/4 tsp salt + more as needed
Freshly ground black pepper to taste
10 g fresh basil leaves chopped (optional)

Cook the shallots, ginger, and garlic in the beet broth in a medium skillet over moderate heat for 4 minutes, stirring.

Stir in the tomatoes and the maple, and gently simmer, stirring occasionally, for 15 minutes.

Season to taste with salt and pepper.

Put the sauce through a blender until smooth puree. Toss with chopped basil.

Serve immediately.

"LOVE IS THE APPETIZER, KNOWLEDGE IS THE MAIN DISH,
AND SEVA (SELFLESS EFFORT FOR THE WELFARE OF ALL) IS THE EXERCISE.
WITHOUT LOVE AND SEVA, KNOWLEDGE BECOMES INDIGESTIBLE"

- GURUDEV SRI SRI RAVI SHANKAR

LENTIL CRISPBREADS

Time - 10 min prep + 45 min baking

Serves - makes 2 trays

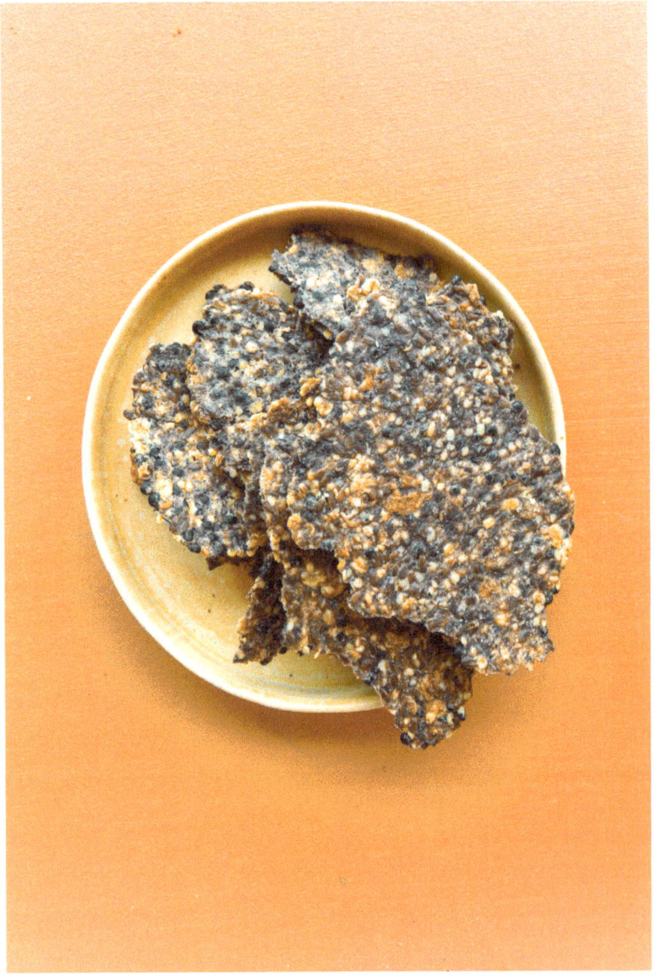

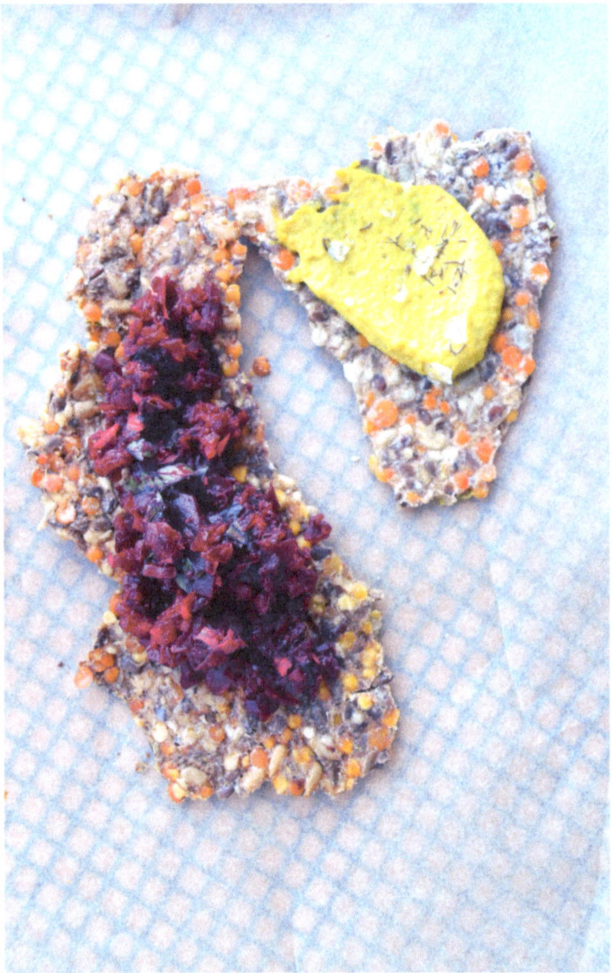

BELUGA WITH HEMP, OAT AND SEEDS

65 g beluga lentils
50 g hemp hearts
60 g gluten-free rolled oats
60 g gluten-free oat flour
50 g flaxseeds
2 tbsp almond butter
2 tbsp chia
1/2 tsp salt
2 tbsp porcini broth or tamari
2 tbsp psyllium husk powder
200 ml hot water

RED LENTIL WITH SUNFLOWER SEEDS AND OAT

125 g red lentils
65 g sunflower seeds
50 g flaxseeds
65 g rolled oats
130 g oat flour
2 tbsp chopped rosemary
2 tbsp chia
1.5 tbsp psyllium husk powder
1/2 tsp salt
2 tbsp chopped fresh rosemary
2 tbsp almond butter
250 ml filtered hot water

If you are making with the red lentils, place them in a bowl cover with the water. Soak overnight, then rinse. For the beluga lentils, no need to soak for long hours. Just soak in warm water for 5-10 minutes, then rinse.

The instruction part is the same for both beluga and red lentil crackers.

Transfer lentils to a large mixing bowl. Add the rest of the ingedients except water. Mix well to combine.

Bring the water to a boil, pour over the dry mixture. Mix until you get a dough-like texture.

Divide the dough in two pieces. Using a rolling pin, roll out until very thin, between two pieces of parchment paper. Divide in two baking trays.

Pre-heat the oven to 150° C with the fan.
Bake the two trays in the oven for 35-40 minutes, then carefully then turn the whole cracker thing around and bake for another 10-12 minutes, until dry and crisp enough.

Let cool for 10 minutes, serve with avocado yogurt dip, beetroot pesto, turmeric hummus (page 32-33) or whatever you like.

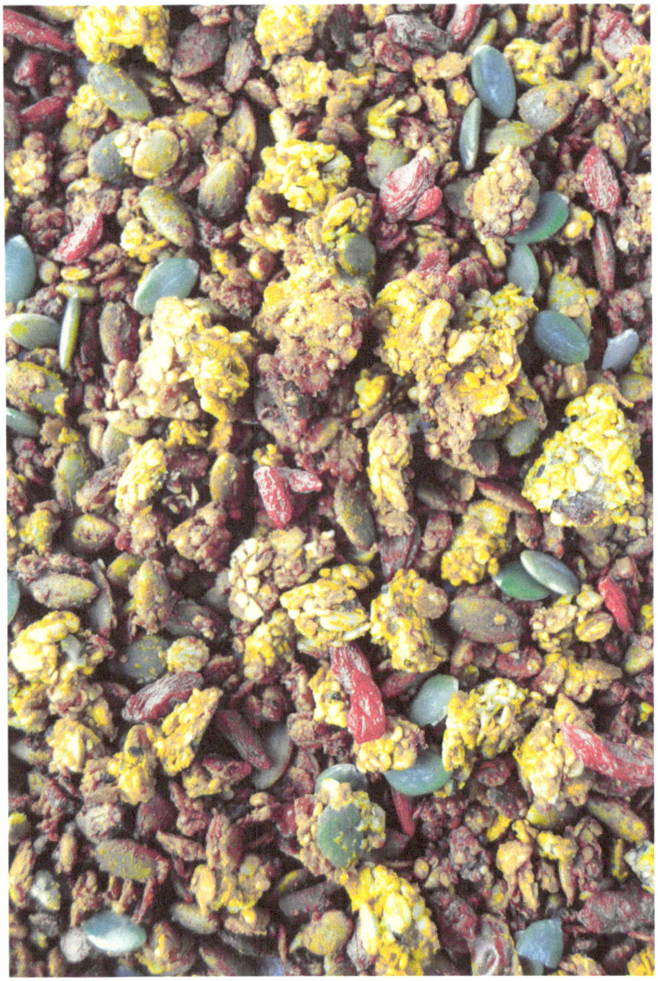

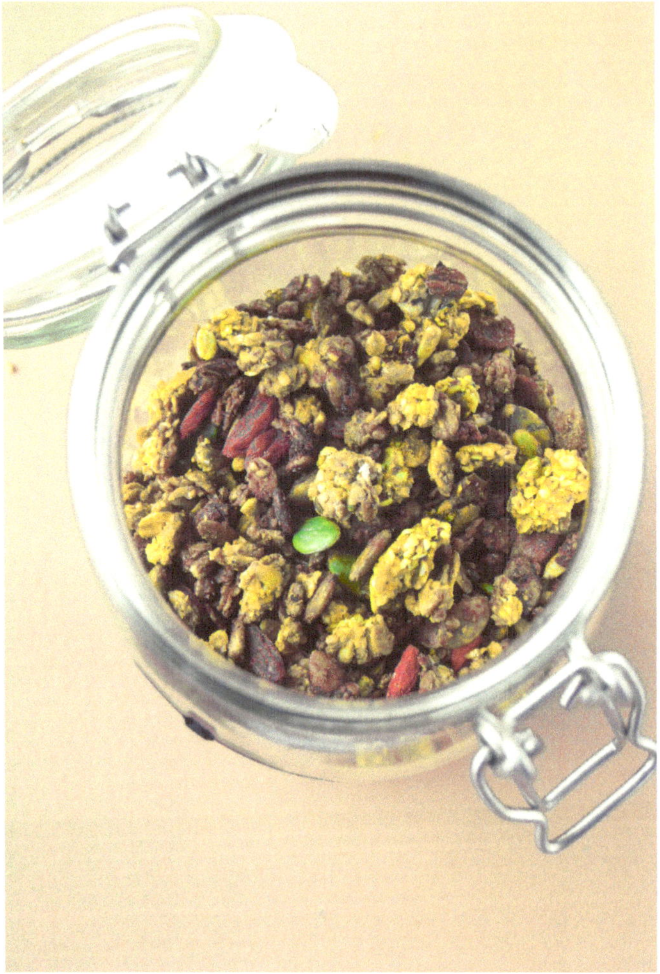

OAT HEMP GRANOLA WITH SEEDS & GOJI

Use on your parfait, yogurt, smoothies or eat on its own for a tasty afternoon snack.

Time - 10 minutes prep + 30 minutes baking
Serves - 1 big batch

200 g rolled oats
120 g pepitas
120 g hemp hearts
65 g sunflower seeds
2 tbsp almond butter
60 g gojiberries
6 fresh sukkari dates + 115 ml water
1 tbsp cinnamon
1/2 tsp cardamom
1/4 tsp salt

Preheat your oven to 175° C.

Mix the oats, sunflower seeds, pepitas, hemp hearts, cinnamon, cardamom and salt.

In a small saucepan, boil the sukkari dates in the water for 35-40 seconds on medium-high heat. Then puree using a spoon, press and stir constantly. Transfer to the mixing bowl.

Using a wooden spoon, mix everything well until every bit gets covered.

Spread out on a baking tray lined parchment paper and toast in the oven until crispy and golden, stirring every 10 minutes, for about 30 minutes.

Once done, add the toasted gojiberries or your favorite dried fruit. Enjoy on your breakfast smoothie, porridge, yogurt or as a snack.

It can be stored up to 2-3 months at room temperature in a airtight glass jar.

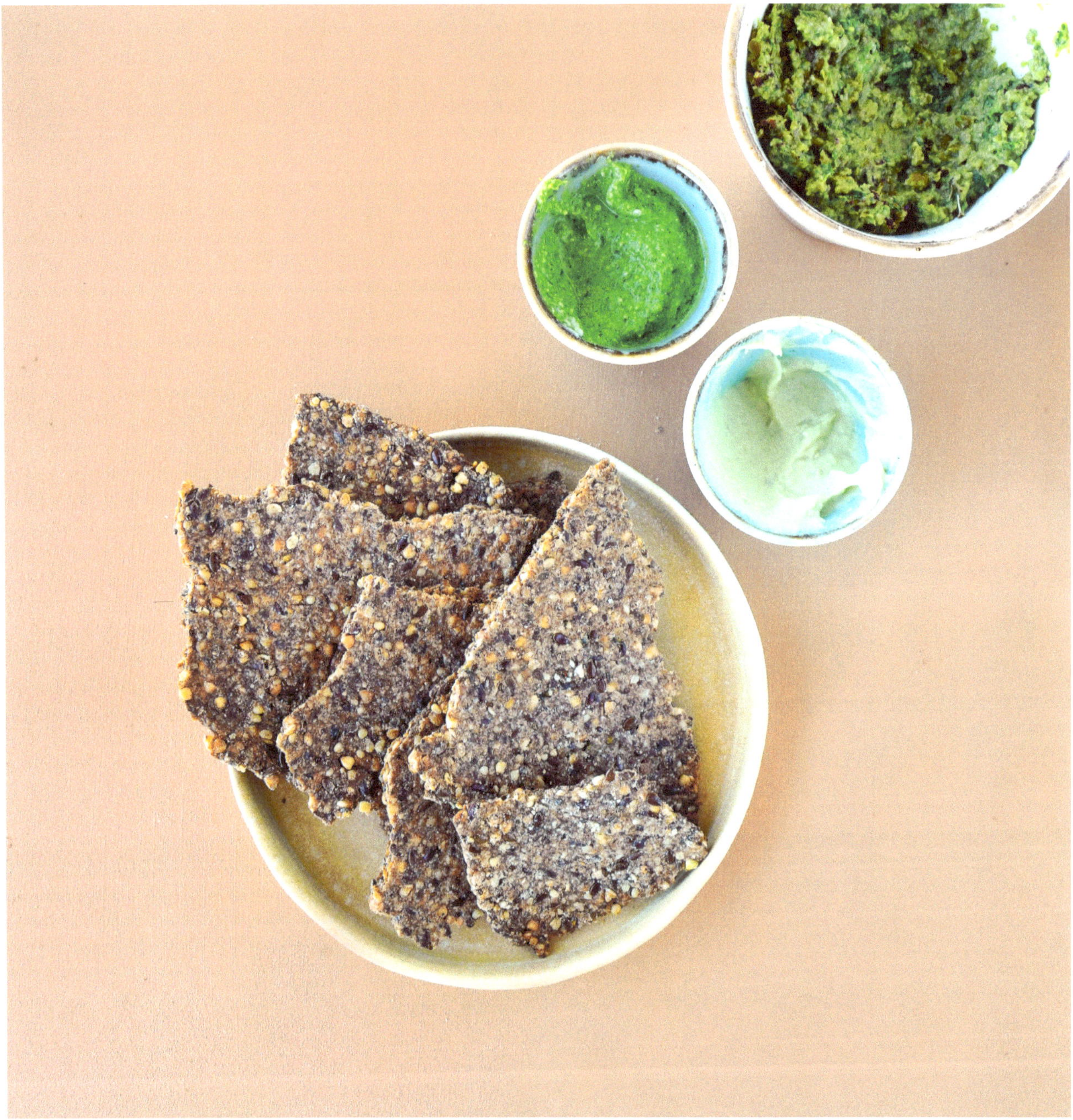

SEEDY BUCKWHEAT CRISPBREAD

This buckwheat crispbread is highly functional as a snack alone or serve them with dip sauces or soup for a filling meal.

Time - 10 min prep + 40 min baking
Serves - makes 2 trays

65 g buckini (soaked dehydrated buckwheat groats)
50 g hemp hearts
50 g almond flour
65 g buckwheat flour
50 g flaxseeds
2 tbsp chia
1/2 tsp salt
2 tbsp almond butter
2 tbsp psyllium husk powder
2 dl hot water

Place the buckinis, hemp hearts, almond flour, buckwheat flour, flaxseeds, chia and salt in a mixing bowl. Mix well.

Then add the almond butter, psyllium husk and hot water. Using a spoon, combine.

Mix until you get a dough-like texture.

Divide the dough in two pieces. Using a rolling pin, roll out until very thin, between two pieces of parchment paper. Divide in two baking trays.

Pre-heat the oven to 150° C with the fan.

Bake the two trays in the oven for 30 minutes, then carefully then turn the whole crispbread thing around and bake for another 10 minutes, until dry and crisp enough.

Let cool for 10 minutes, serve with roasted carrot soup or enjoy as it is.

ROASTED CARROT TOMATO SOUP WITH FENNEL

Time - 35 minutes

Serves - 4 person

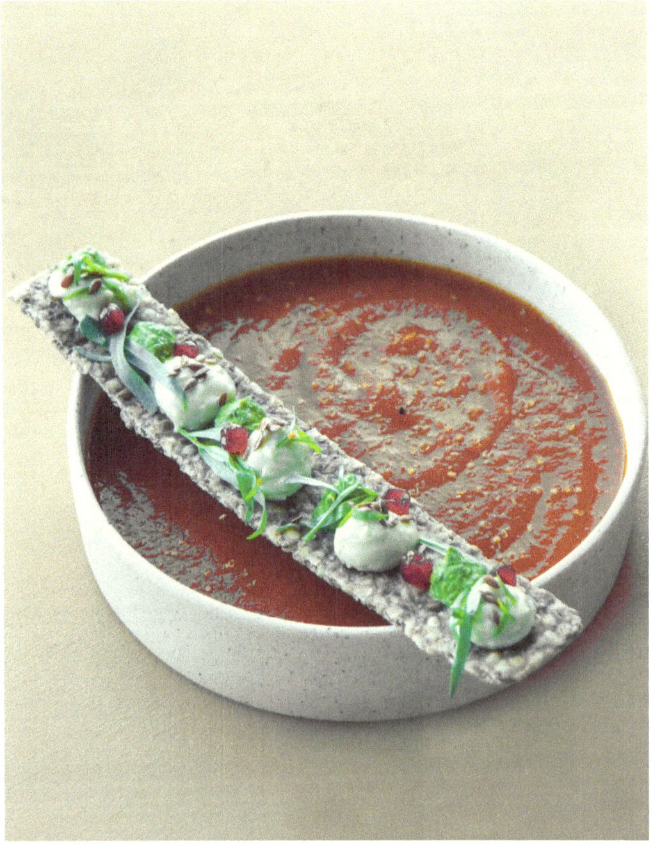

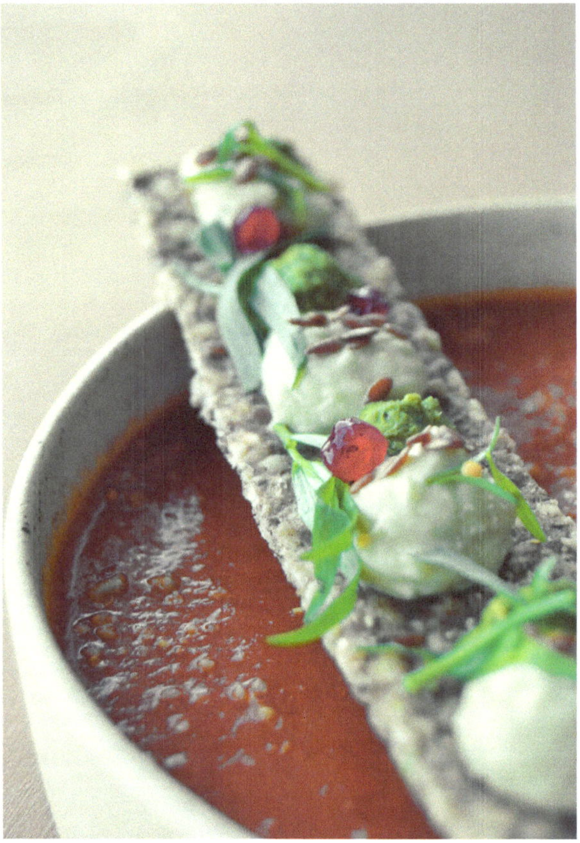

This delicious carrot soup flavoured with earthy fennel, served with buckwheat crispbread, dandelion pesto, onion cream, fresh tarragon and lingonberries.

200 g tomatoes
300 g carrots
2 red bell pepper
2 sweet onion chopped
2 garlic cloves minced
4 cups white vegetable broth
4 tbsp beetroot broth to saute
40 g fennel bulb chopped
1/4 cup chopped fennel
1 bay leaf
Lemon juice to serve

To serve (optional)
Buckwheat crispbread (page 45)
Dandelion pesto (page 35)
Onion cream (page 61)
Lingonberries (or other forest fruits)
Fresh tarragon

Preheat oven to 205° C. Line a large baking sheet with parchment paper.

Peel and cut the carrots into 1/2-inch rounds. On a baking sheet, toss the carrots and celery bulb with 2 tablespoons of the beet broth and sprinkle generously with salt. Roast the carrots and fennel until they become brown and soften, turning them over with a spatula every 10 minutes or so; this should take 15 to 20 minutes.

Put the onion in a medium stock pot with the remaining beet broth. Brown the onion over medium heat, stirring frequently. Add the garlic, chopped red bell pepper, tomatoes, fennel and then add the carrots. Cook on medium heat for 2-3 minutes.

Add the vegetable broth and bay leaf. Bring to boil and simmer for 5 to 10 minutes, until the carrots and peppers are soft enough to puree. Once cooked remove the bay leaf from the mixture.

Use an immersion or a standard blender to puree the mixture until smooth. If the soup seems too thick, add more stock or water and reheat gently. Add salt and pepper to taste.

For a gourmet effect, serve with buckwheat crispbread cut lengthwise topped onion cream, lingon and lemon wedges. Use a piping bag and squeeze the creams on the crispbread to decorate if desired.

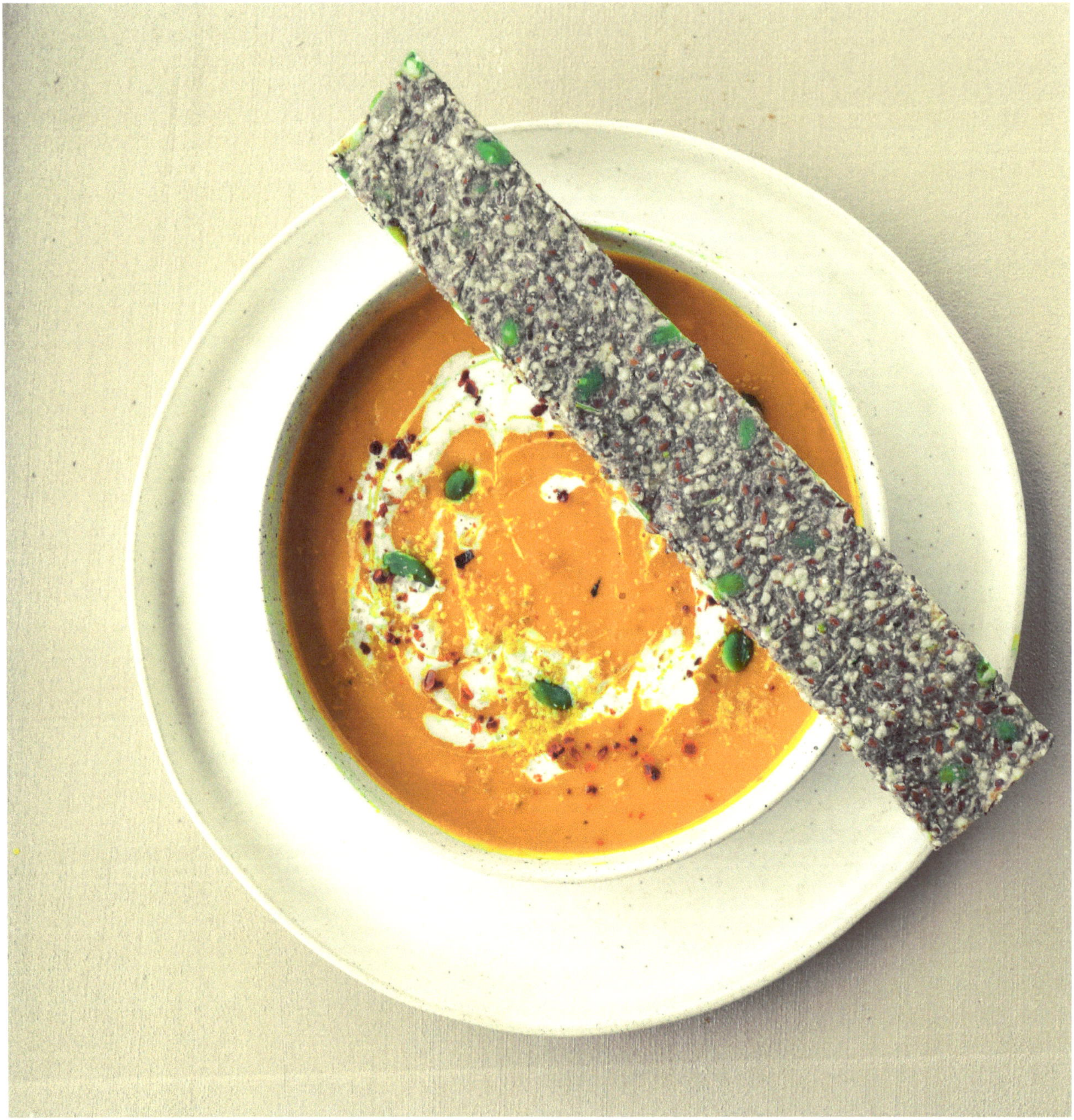

PUMPKIN SOUP

This soup is warming, creamy and packed with autumnal flavours - ready in 25 minutes using stovetop.

Time - 10 min prep + 15 min cooking
Serves - 4 person

1 kg acorn squash or pumpkin of your choice, chopped weight after peeled and removed seeds
2 large white onions chopped
4 garlic cloves minced
4 tbsp white vegetable broth
500 ml water
100 ml almond milk
1 tsp salt
1/4 tsp ground nutmeg
1 tsp red pepper flakes

To serve
Buckwheat crispbread (page 45, just replace buckini with pumpkin seeds)
Pumpkin seeds for garnish
Extra red pepper flakes
Onion cream (page 61), (or other plant-based creams like coconut, oat, almond etc.) to serve (optional)

Heat the vegetable broth in a large pot. Add the garlic and onion and cook over medium-high heat until golden brown, stirring occasionally.
Add the pumpkin and cook for another 2-3 minutes, stirring occasionally.
Incorporate all the remaining ingredients and bring to a boil, then cook over medium-high heat for about 15 minutes or until the pumpkin is tender.
Blend the mixture in a blender. Add more or less liquid depending on how thick you want your soup to be.

Serve with pumpkin seeds, coconut cream and pumpkin seed cracker if desired.
Keep the leftovers in an airtight container in the fridge for 5 days.

TIPS - Customize your soup with any ingredient you'd like. The recipe goes well with veggies like leeks, carrots, cauliflower, potatoes or celery in the place of pumpkins (in case they are not in the season), or with spices like ground cinnamon, nutmeg, or cayenne powder

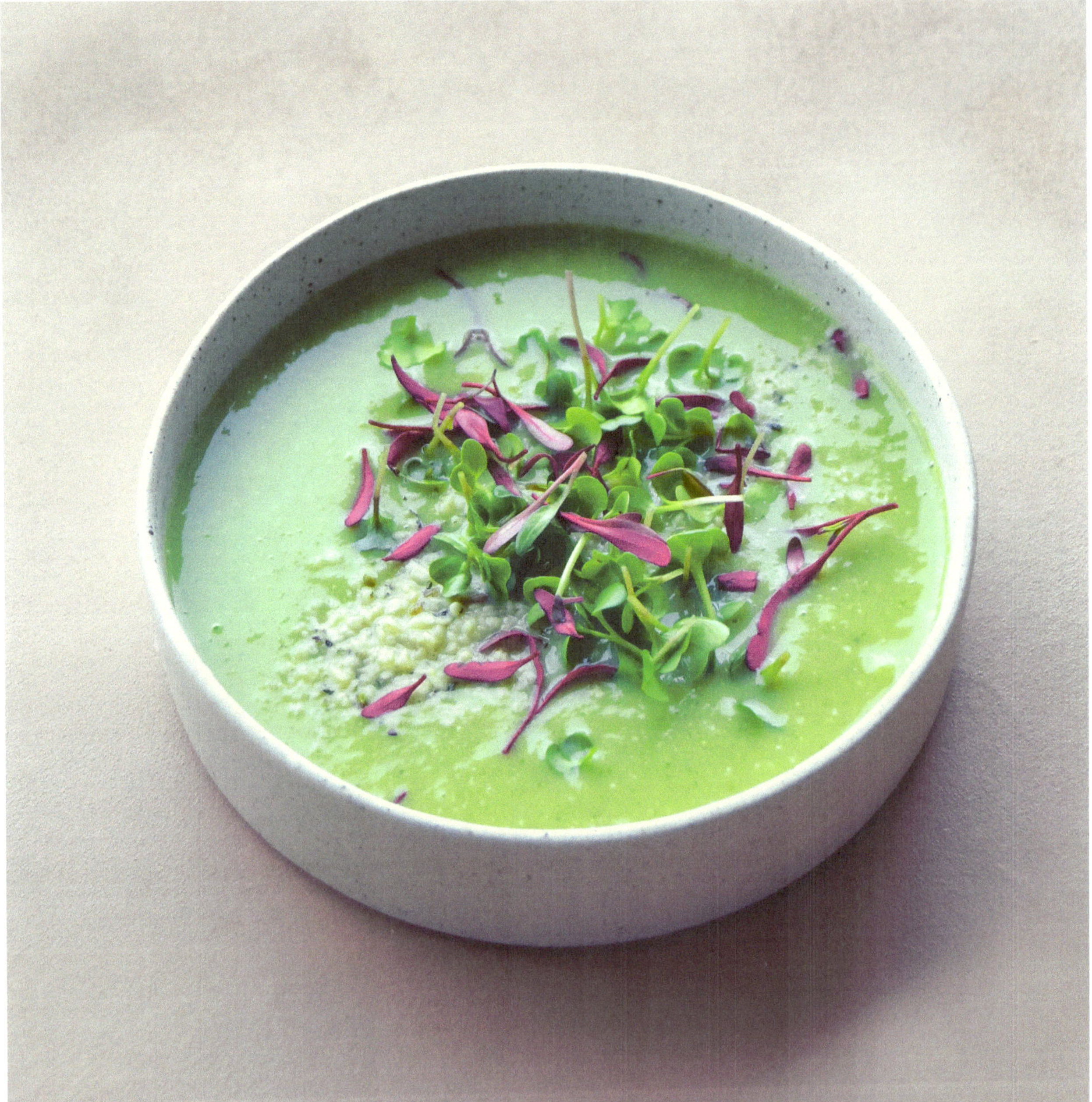

BROCCOLI SOUP WITH GINGER

This delicious ginger flavoured broccoli soup packed with nutritious microgreens and hemp hearts. Also can be made with the cauliflower in the place of broccoli or carrots and zucchini together when broccoli is not in the season.

Time - 20 minutes
Serves - 4 person

400 g broccoli
1 large red onion
2 garlic cloves minced
1/4 cup beetroot broth
20 g fresh ginger
600 ml filtered water
1 tsp salt
1 tsp spirulina powder (optional)
Radish and beetroot microgreens to serve
Hemp hearts to serve
Lemon wedges to serve

Peel your ginger, onion and garlic, chop finely. Place in a large pot. Pour the beetroot broth. Cook on medium heat until onions are soften enough and nicely caramelized in the beet broth.

Wash your broccoli, drain, trim and cut the stalk in half, then finely slice it. Add to your pot. Toss well with the onions, garlic and ginger. Then add the filtered water and cook for 8-10 minutes, or until tender – you should be able to poke the tip of a knife easily into the florets.

Once done, let it cool for 5-6 minutes. Then transfer to your blender. Add the spirulina, and more water if you need.Blend until silky smooth.
Pour back in the pot. Heat on low heat for about 2-3 minutes. Immediately serve with lemon wedges, garnish with micro-greens and sprinkle some hemp hearts for a nutritious soup packed with omega.

Serve with lentil crackers or buckwheat bread for a filling meal.

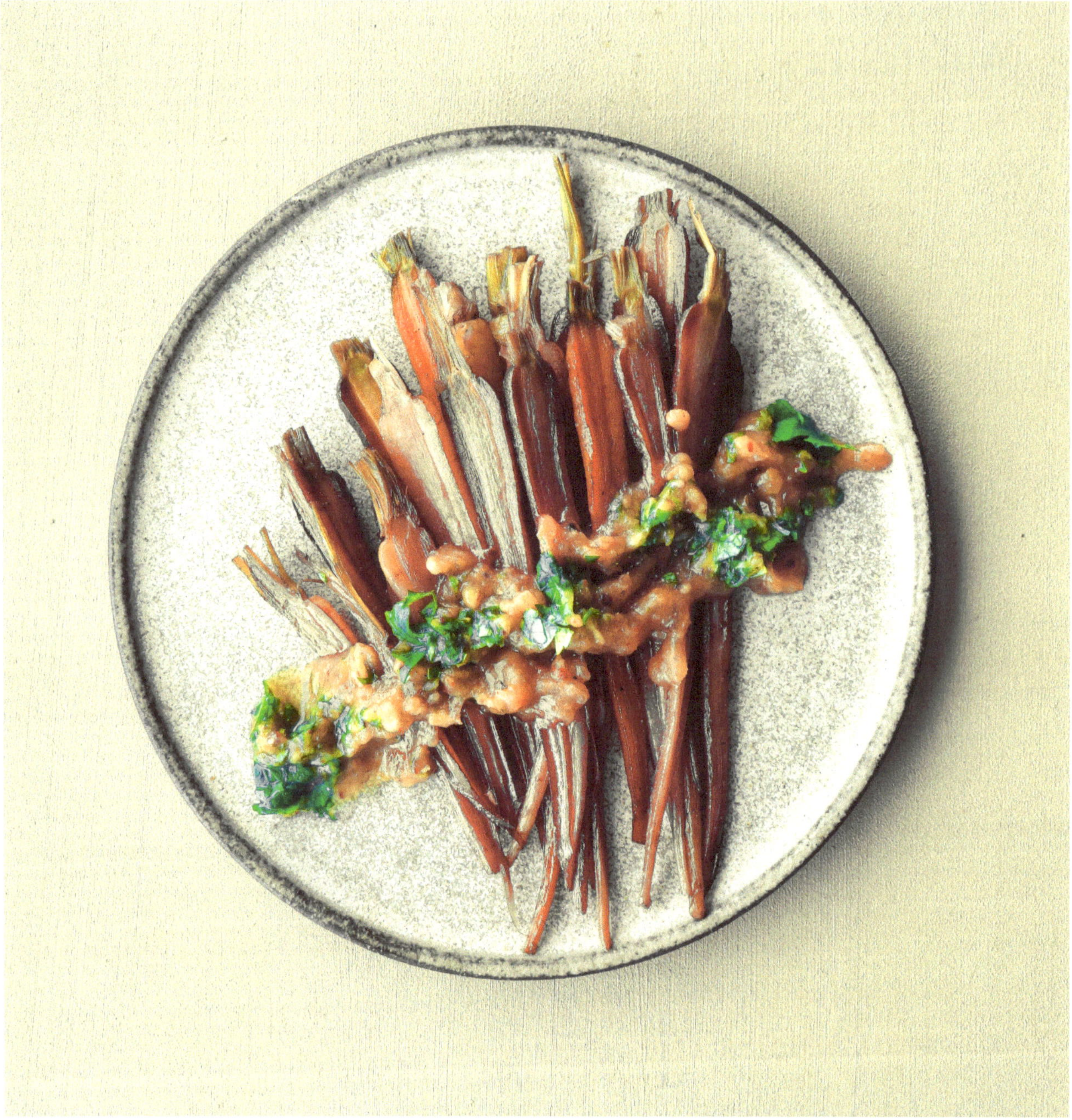

ROASTED PARSNIPS WITH TAMARIND GINGER DRESSING

Tamarind is a bit like a date in flavour, only with a much tarter finish. Combined with spices, chilli, ginger and lime it make tangy, sharp sauce that works beautifully with the caramelised sweetness of roasted parsnips.

Time - 1 hour
Serves - 2-3 person as a side

300 g colorful parsnips peeled and cut in half

Tamarind Ginger Dressing

4 fresh tamarind peeled seeds removed
3 fresh sukkari date, seeds removed
1 tbsp balsamic vinegar
2 tbsp chopped fresh parsley
1 tsp red chili flakes
4 g finely chopped or grated ginger
Juice of 1 lemon
Salt and pepper to taste

Preheat oven to 190° C.
Put the parsnips in a baking dish and toss in just enough balsamic to coat. Season well. Roast for 45 minutes-1 hour, until tender and browned (caramelised bits are a good thing with parsnips).

Place the tamarind, dates, balsamic, grated ginger, lemon juice and chili in the blender, blitz until smooth.
Add a pinch salt and more pepper if you need. Taste and arrange the flavour.

Wash, drain and chop some fresh parsley.

When parsnips are done, transfer to a serving plate.

Top with tamarind dressing, sprinkle some chopped parsley. Serve with your main dish. This side dish is also great in buddha bowls.

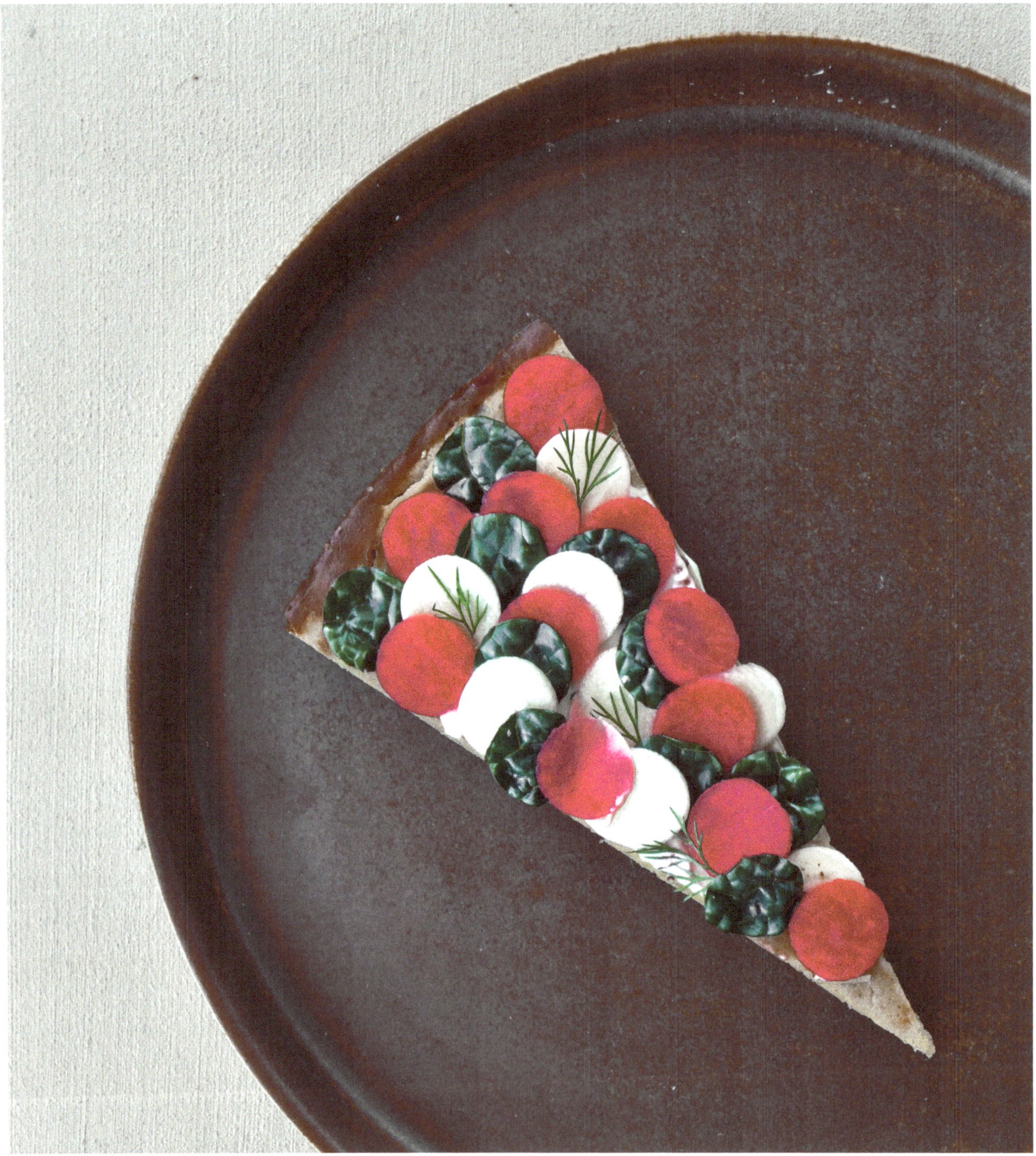

HARLEQUIN FARINATA

A savory and custardy chickpea pancake from Italy, served with sunflower seed cream, colorful greens and roots.

Time - 55 minutes
Serves - 4

150 g sprouted chickpea flour
250 ml lukewarm water
1 tbsp smooth sunflower butter (or almond butter)
3 springs of green onion chopped
Salt and black pepper to taste

Toppings
4-5 leaves cavolo nero
1 kohlrabi or courgette
1 watermelon radish
3-4 tbsp apple cider vinegar
Fresh dill
Capers (optional)
Sunflower seed cream (page 161)

Preheat the oven to 220° C on the grill setting.

To make the farinata batter, put the chickpea flour, chopped green onions, water, a teaspoon of salt, a generous grind of black pepper and the sunflower seed butter in a large mixing bowl. Whisk until well combined then set aside to thicken for 20 minutes. Make sure to use lukewarm water so the chickpea flour dissolves well. Once done, pour batter on a baking tray lined parchment paper. Bake the batter for approximately 30 to 35 minutes until it is golden brown and crispy on top.

Meanwhile, to make the harlequin toppings, slice the kohlrabi and watermelon radish very thinly using a mandolin slicer. Wash and drain your cavolo nero. Using a small round cutter, cut the cavolo nero leaves, kohlrabi and watermelon radish into small rounds. Place in a bowl, drizzle with apple cider vinegar, set it for 10 minutes.

Cut the farinata into wedges. Spread sunflower seed cream over farinata, top with harlequin rounds, garnish with fresh dill and capers if desired. Serve as a starter or with a green salad for a lunch or dinner.

To store, place the farinata in an airtight container and store it in the refrigerator for up to 5 days. Reheat it in the stove oven for 5 minutes before eating.

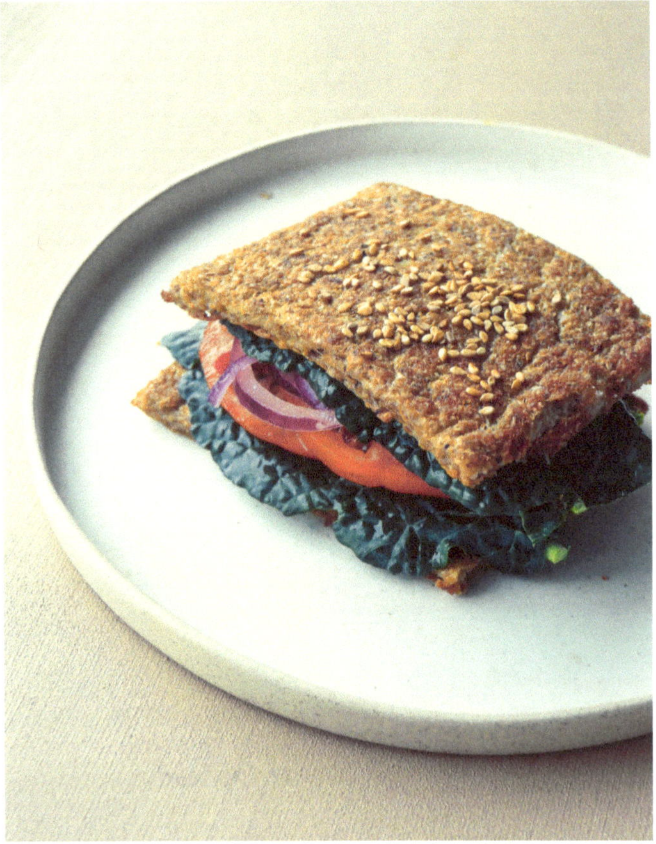

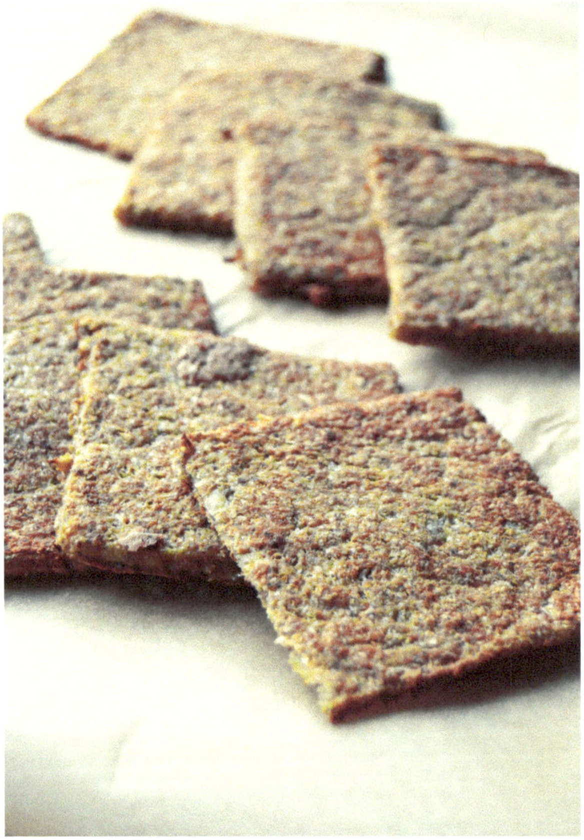

CAULIFLOWER FLAT BREAD

My new favorite cauliflower bread is so delicious and healthy - made with whole cauliflower florets and chickpea flour. So easy to make and addictive!

Time - 10 min prep + 25 min baking
Makes - 10 slices

600 g cauliflower florets
75 g sprouted chickpea flour
50 g almond flour
50 g cassava or tapioca
2 tbsp psyllium husk
1-2 tbsp water
1 tsp dried herbs of your choice
Salt and pepper to taste

Filling
Cavolo nero or your favorite greens
Thinly sliced tomatoes
Thinly sliced red onion
Avocado mayonnaise or hemp ranch sauce (page 19-20)

Preheat the oven to 200° C.
Line a baking tray with parchment paper.
Wash, drain and chop your cauliflower, place in the food processor. Process until fine rice-like texture. Then transfer to a larger mixing bowl.
Then add the chickpea flour, water, psyllium husk powder, cassava, salt, pepper and herbs.
Stir well to combine together. Let it sit for 2-3 minutes until you get a sticky dough. Then lightly knead with your hands in the bowl. (Depending on the water content of your cauliflower, you may need to add more water. Please carefully check the consistency after 2-3 minutes sitting and kneading, if necessary add one more tbsp water.) Once the dough is sticky, transfer to the parchment paper and form into a rectangular. Roll out between two parchment paper gently. Remove the top parchment and bake for 25-30 minutes or until slightly golden and firm enough.
Remove from the oven and let cool completely at least 15 minutes.
Turn it upside-down and carefully remove the baking paper. Cut into bread-sized slices. Make sandwich with simple kale leaves, red onion and tomatoes as I did if you want.
You can also roll them into wraps with your favorite filling, make bite size canapés, buns (page 137) or enjoy alone.

If you want to use less cauliflower, you can swap 200 g cauliflower with carrots and use 400 g cauliflower.
The recipe also can be made with broccoli florets but I found cauliflower one more tastier.

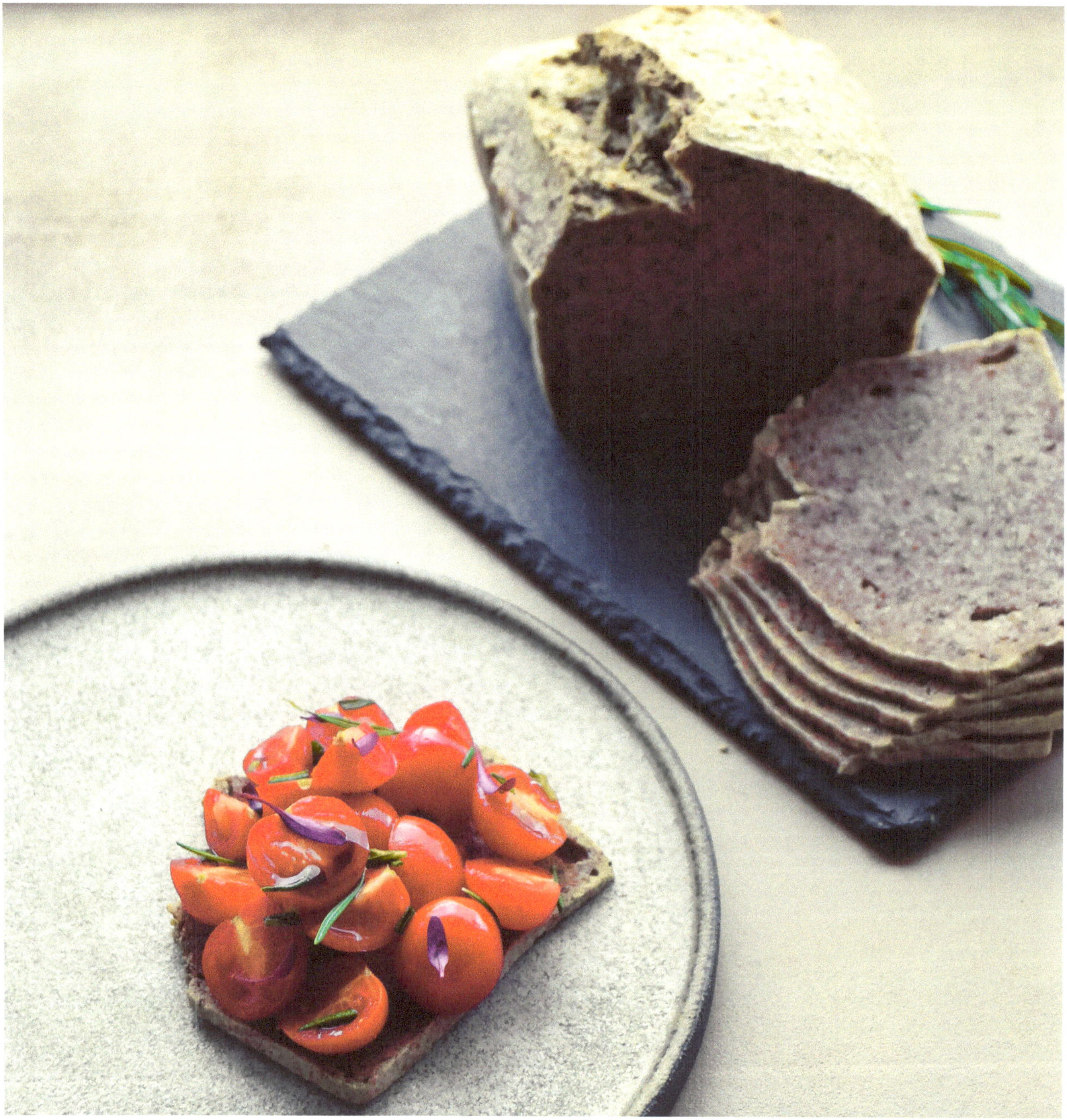

YEAST-FREE BUCKWHEAT BREAD

Highly nutritious whole grain bread that is naturally gluten-free and a good source of protein, fiber, and energy.

Time - 15 min prep + 90 min baking
Makes - 22x12 cm loaf

500 g unroasted buckwheat groats soaked for 30 minutes, strained and rinsed
2 tbsp chia seeds + 6 tbsp water
1 tsp salt
1 tsp baking soda
1 cup filtered water

TIPS - Depending on your oven, you may need to bake the bread slightly longer or shorter. To test the bread, stick a toothpick in it. If the toothpick comes out clean, the bread is cooked. This bread is meant to be denser than a regular wheat loaf of bread. Store this bread in the fridge. Toast before eating for the best taste.
If you like airy texture, let the buckwheats sit after blending process in a warm place for about 12-14 hours before baking process. As I don't prefer fermentation, baked it directly.

Whisk the chia seeds and water together in a bowl. Set aside for for 10 minutes or until it becomes gelly.
Preheat the oven to 160° C and line a 22 x12 cm loaf pan with parchment paper.
Place the soaked rinsed buckwheat groats, filtered water, baking soda and salt together in a food processor or blender. Then transfer mixture in a mixing bowl.
Add the chia seeds and using a spoon mix until everything is well combined.
Spoon the sticky dough evenly into your loaf pan.
Bake for 1 hour 30 minutes, until the bread is firm to touch. Using a toothpick, check if it is completely cooked. The crust will be softer when you bake at low temperature for long hours.

Once cooked, remove from the oven and let cool for 15 minutes, before removing the bread from the pan and allowing to cool completely on a wire rack.

Once cooled, slice thinly. This bread is the best when sliced very thinly. When you refrigerate bread overnight, it will be very easy to cut thinly with a chef knife. Slightly fry both sides of the thin slices in a non-stick pan or bread toaster before serving.
Store the cooled bread in an airtight container at cool room temperature for 2 days, in the refrigerator for 1 week, and the freezer for up to 6 months.

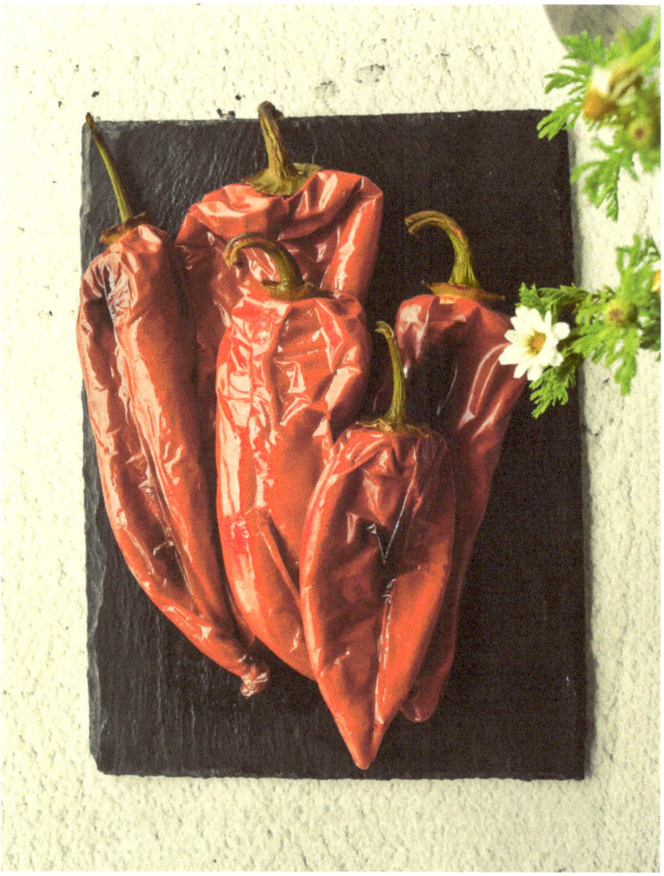

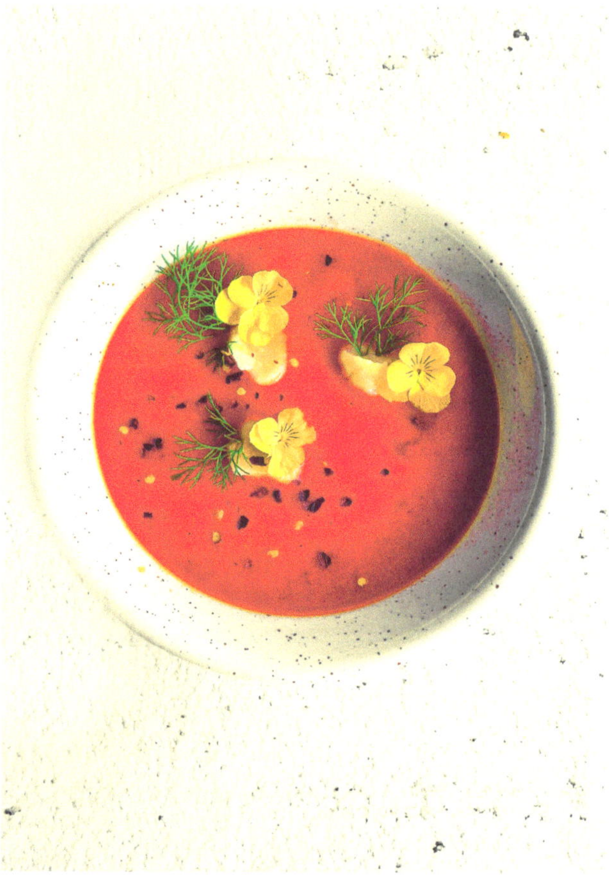

ROASTED RED BELL PEPPER SOUP

This delicious red bell pepper soup is enhanced with onion cream and takes it a level further. If you do not have any issue with the onions, you can use cream of onion as a cream alternative in all your soups.

Time - 80 minutes
Serves - 2 person

400 g red bell peppers
200 g san marzano tomatoes cut in half
600 ml water or veg stock + more if you need
2 tbsp fresh dill
1 tbsp roasted garlic puree
A pinch red chili flakes
2-3 tbsp onion cream to serve
Viola to decorate

Onion Cream
3 large vidalia onions*
1 tbsp lemon juice
Black pepper, chili or chipotle to season (optional)

Roast red peppers, tomatoes and garlic at 200° C for 15-20 minutes in the oven on a foil-lined baking sheet until tender and charred on all sides.
Then remove red peppers, tomatoes and garlic from the oven, let cool to the touch, and remove charred outer skin seeds and stems. Transfer to a high speed blender and add water to purée soup. (If you prefer, you can also use the seeds and skins too, they are nutritious and delicious.)

Then transfer back to pot and bring to a simmer over medium-low heat. Taste and adjust seasonings as needed.
Let simmer on low for at least 10 more minutes. The longer it simmers, the deeper the flavor develops.
Serve as is or top with desired toppings, we used fresh dill, chili flakes, viola and onion cream.

To make onion cream, roast the onions with their peels at 200° C in a roasting pan that fits them snugly for about 50 minutes, or until they are very dark on the outside and molten soft on the inside. Let them cool for 15-20 minutes.

Once they have cooled, Remove the peels, and add the onions into a high speed blender. (Food processor doesn't give you the same results.) Blend until very smooth, about 1 to 2 minutes. Finish by adding freshly squeezed lemon juice, then blend 20 seconds more. Adjust seasoning if necessary. Chipotle, chili or black pepper goes well together.

roasted red bell pepper soup continued

To store the sauce: Keep in the fridge for up to 2-3 days, or freeze for up to two weeks. In either case, blend in the blender for 20 to 30 seconds to reincorporate just before serving.

Glossary

*Vidalia Onions are the most common kinds of sweet onions. They are fairly similar to yellow onions in flavor, though their layers are slightly less tender and meaty.

Extremely low in pyruvic acid—which, when exposed to air, makes your eyes tear—Vidalias are among the mildest in the onion kingdom.

How to Shop and Store: Vidalia onion season typically runs from the middle of April through early September. Firm, medium-sized onions without any bruises will taste the best. To store the onions, wrap each onion in a paper towel and store in the fridge; they'll keep for weeks.

Caramelize onions in the pan without olive oil

You probably heard that caramelizing heats the onion so high that the sugars begin to release fast and create with new depth of flavor you're looking for. This sounds like it's going to be complicated. No way! The natural sugar in an onion requires no frying but patience. I may add a sprinkle of nutmeg or black pepper but no salt, sugar or oil.

Instructions

Slice onions into thin shreds.

Place slices into a uniform layer on a nonstick pan on medium heat and cover with water, beet stock or mushroom stock just to the top of the onions. Cook until water is absorbed.

When foamy water is boiling out of the onions and they appear dry add water again to the top layer of onions. Don't stir yet. The idea is to cook out the moisture so you'll see a color change of your onions as this proceeds.

Don't stir the onions until the second water is absorbed. Then add about 2 tbsp of vegetable stock, beet stock or mushroom broth and stir the onions. You will begin to see the caramelization in full effect and gently stir them to loosen up any adherent onions from the bottom keeping heat even. And not turning it up, continue to stir. They will begin to brown and become gooey.

This takes about 15 minutes.

TIPS - A pinch of baking soda can bring out a new taste dimension when browning onions. A small addition of baking soda yields onions which taste remarkably sweet with strong caramel notes.

BLOOMED BLACK WILD RICE TABBOULEH

Time - 12 hr soaking + 15 min prep.

Serves - 2

90 g wild black rice (blackened or wood-parched)
1 cup pomegranate seeds
1 large tomato
1 large red bell pepper
1/4 cup fresh mint leaves
1 cup fresh parsley
1/2 cup fresh dill
1/4 cup green onions
Juice of 1 whole lemon
Salt and pepper to taste

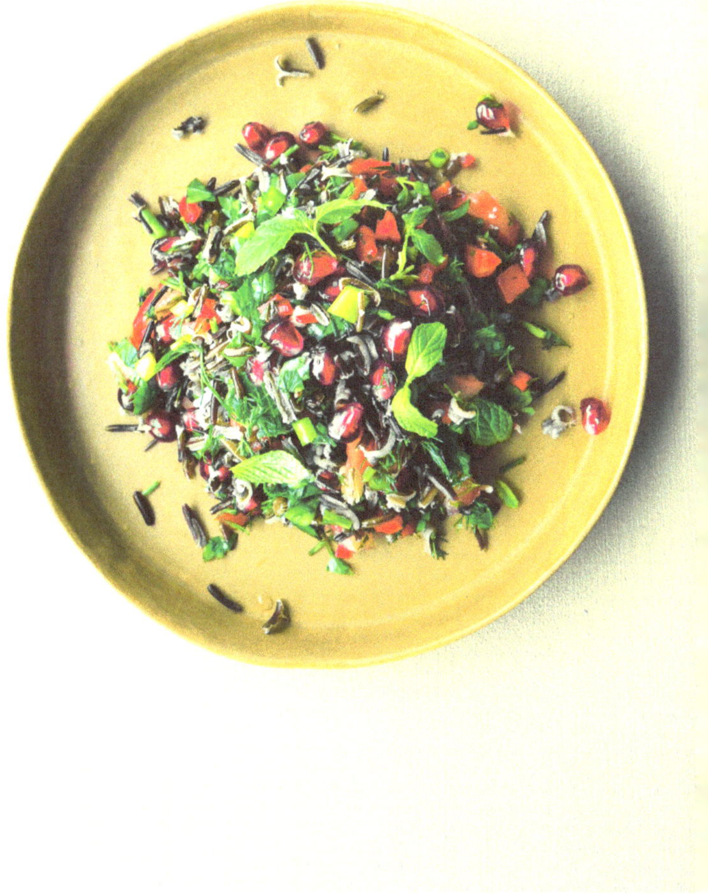

Place the wild black rice in a pot, cover with water. Let it soak at least 12-14 hours or overnight. Then rinse well. Eating any other rice raw is not recommended. Black rice blooms when soaked overnight, and this is why it can be eaten raw. The hard outer shell of the black rice (also known as the hull) will bloom during overnight soaking. Blooming means the rice softens and the hull breaks open exposing the innards of the rice as if it were cooked. So even though it's raw, it has the texture of being cooked.
Chop your herbs finely, cut the red bell pepper and tomato into small cubes.
In a large mixing bowl, mix all bloomed rice with the rest of the ingredients together. Give them a good toss. Taste, adjust the salt and pepper.

TIPS - You can also use cooked quinoa or rolled oats in the place of black wild rice, if you prefer.

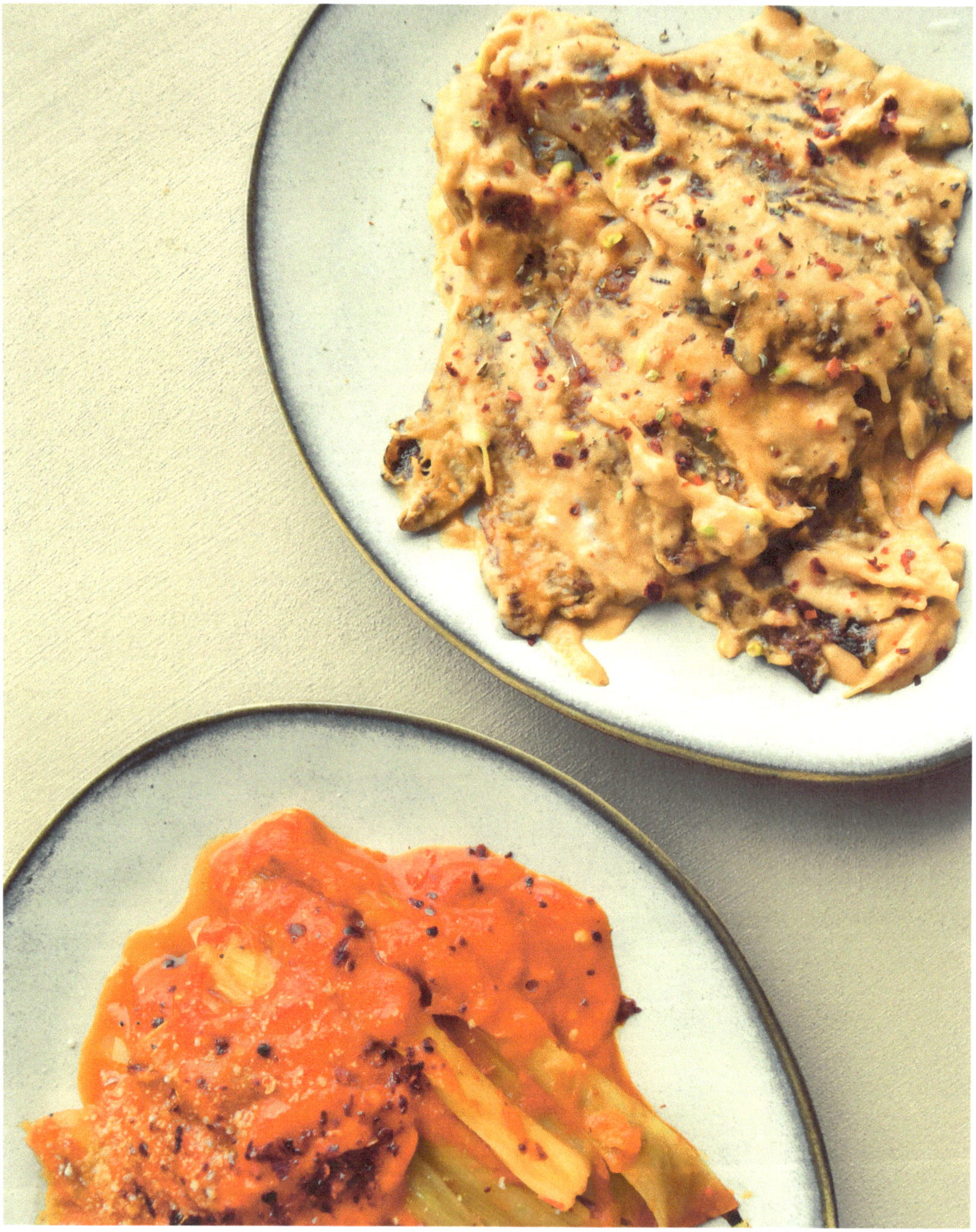

ROASTED LEEKS WITH ROMESCO SAUCE

Time - 50 minutes
Serves - 2

2 red bell peppers cut in half and deseeded
2 large tomato cut in half
40 g toasted almonds
1 medium yellow onion
1 garlic clove chopped
2 tsp sherry vinegar
1/4 tsp paprika
4 leeks cut in half lengthwise
60 ml white vegetable broth

Preheat oven to 230° C. Line a baking tray with parchment paper, place the bell peppers (skin-side up), tomatoes, onion and garlic. Bake for 25 minutes or until the peppers begin to colour. Let it cool.

In a high speed blender, add the peppers, tomato, onions and garlic, veg broth with the almonds, paprika, and vinegar, purée until smooth. Season with salt and pepper. Set aside.

Place the leeks cut-side down in a deep pot. Cook for 15 minutes or until tender. Then brown under a preheated grill for 5 minutes or until golden.

Spread half the Romesco sauce over the bottom of a serving platter. Place the leeks cut-side up in the sauce. Serve with the remaining sauce on the top.

OYSTER MUSHROOMS WITH BUTTER BEAN MASH AND PICADA SAUCE

Time - 70 minutes
Serves - 2

200 g oyster mushrooms
4 garlic cloves minced
1 red onion chopped
4 tbsp beetroot broth
1 tbsp tomato paste
1/2 tsp chili flakes
1/2 tsp coriander powder
1 tsp salt
1 cup butter bean mash (page 34)
1/2 cup picada sauce (page 36)

Preheat oven to 150° C fan.

In a large bowl, combine the mushrooms, beet broth, garlic, onion, chili, coriander, tomato paste, and salt and stir to mix.

Place mixture in a cooking bag, tie the bag with a string and place on a baking tray.

Cook for 40 minutes, once done flip the bag and return to the oven for 20 minutes more, or until the mushrooms are very tender.

Then transfer to a mixing bowl, add the butter bean mash and picada sauce over the mushrooms, toss well.

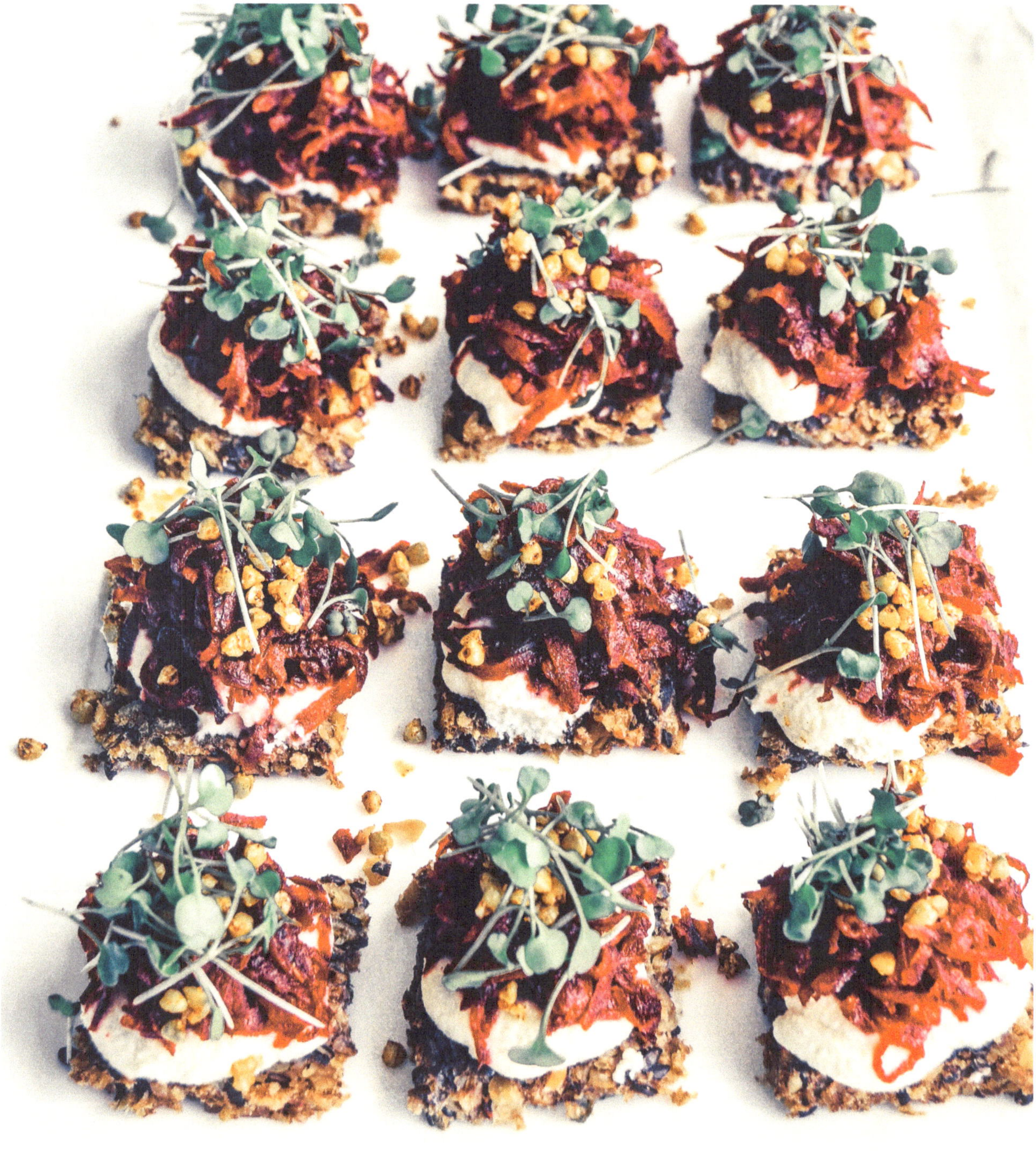

BEETROOT CANAPES

For a quick and easy bite-size snack, serve buckwheat bread cut in small squares to make canapés, top with beet, almond cream, microgreens and spicy buckinis.

Time - 50 minutes
Serves - 24 small bites

6-7 thinly sliced yeast-free buckwheat bread (page 59)
1 cup broccoli microgreens
70 g buckini (activated and dehydrated buckwheat groats)
1/4 tsp chili pepper
1/4 tsp salt

Marinated beetroots
2 large beetroots
1 small golden apple
40 ml balsamic vinegar
1 garlic cloves minced
1/2 tsp salt

Almond cheese cream
130 g almonds soaked
3 garlic cloves minced
1/8 tsp black pepper
1/2 tsp salt
1/2 cup water + more as needed
4 tbsp lemon juice
1 tsp dijon mustard

To preapre the beetroots, in a large bowl, shred the beetroots and apples.
Add the balsamic, salt and garlic cloves. Stir together.
Let it sit for 20-25 minutes to develop the flavour.

Meanwhile, soak your almonds in warm water for 15 minutes. Once they are soften enough, peel their skin. Remove the skin and water. Then add the peeled almonds to your blender. (You can also use blanched almonds if you want to make the process easier.)

Add the minced garlic, salt, mustard and water in the blender. Blend until smooth and creamy, scraping down as you go. Add more water a little at a time if necessary. If you want a thicker cheese, start with 2 tbsp of water and add more as needed.

Then add the lemon juice and blend to incorporate. Taste and add more salt and lemon juice if desired.

In a small bowl, mix the buckini, chili pepper and salt well.

To assemble, spread almond cheese on the top of bread bites, serve along with the marinated beetroot apple mixture, spicy buckini and microgreens.

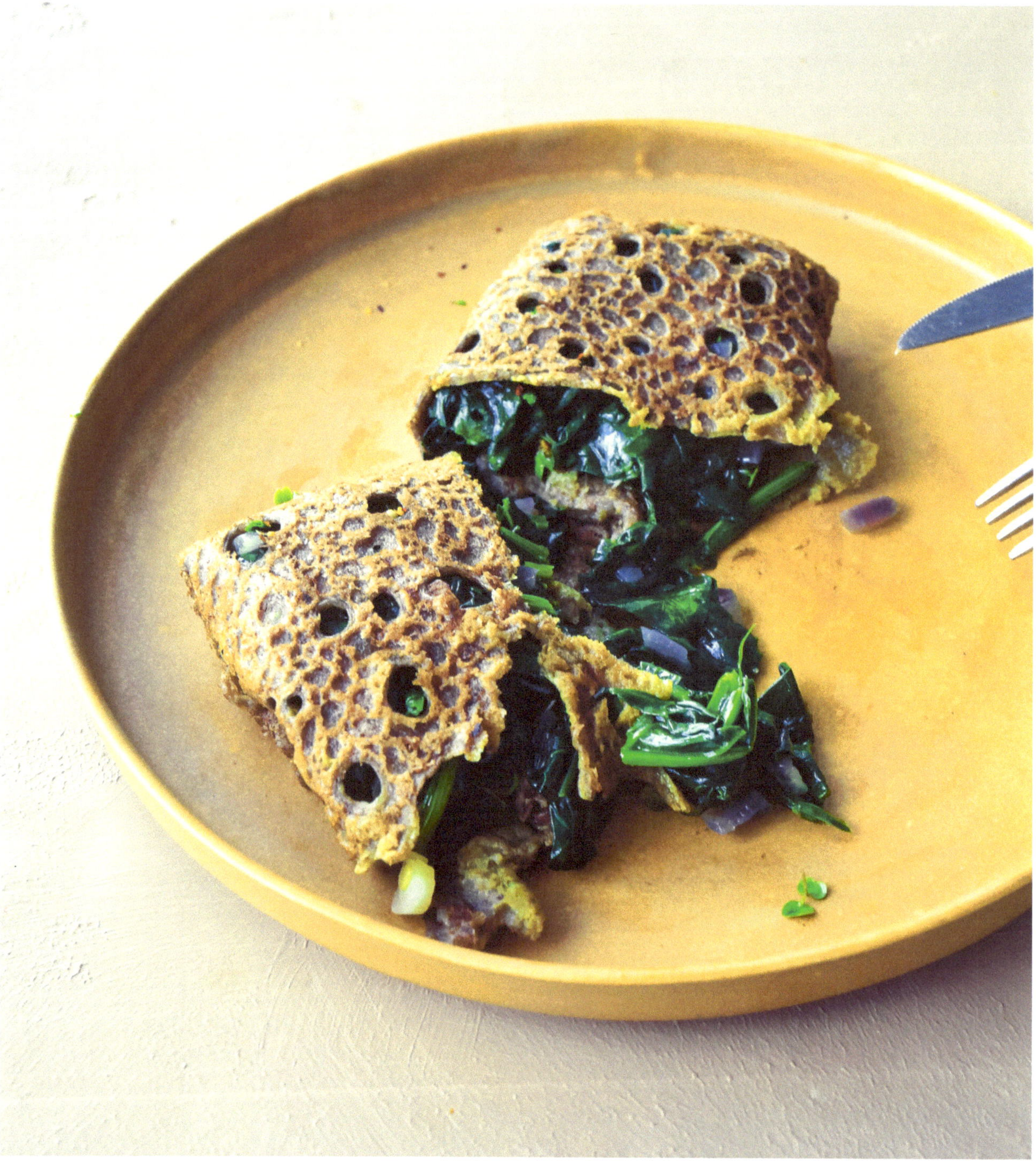

BUCKWHEAT CREPES WITH SPINACH FILLING

These buckwheat crepes have a distinct flavor that can be a little intense with buckwheat flour. It's earthy and nutty, with a slightly bitter edge, if you prefer, you can reduce the buckwheat ratio and add some oat flour.

Time - 10 min prep + 15 min baking
Serves - 2-3

100 g buckwheat flour
250 ml oat milk
1 tsp baking powder
1 tsp salt

Spinach Filling
1 red onion chopped
3 garlic cloves
400g spinach
1/4 tsp blackpepper
Salt to taste
1/4 cup vegetable broth

Place sprouted buckwheat flour, baking powder and salt in a mixing bowl, mix well.
Then add the oat milk, stir well. You need to get a thin pancake batter consistency.

Preheat a large non-stick pan over medium-high heat.
Pour one ladle mixture over the pan. Move the pan around until the batter evenly covers the bottom of the pan.

Cook for about one minute or until the batter gets darker, loosen the edges with a spatula and flip the crepe.

Repeat the process until you've used up all the remaining batter.

To make spinach filling, place the onions, garlic and vegetable broth in the pan, cook until soften. Then add the washed, drained fresh spinach, toss well.
On the medium heat, stirring constantly cook them for 1-2 minutes until bright green Then add salt and black pepper.
Serve with the crepes.

Best when consumed immediately, they can also be covered and stored in the refrigerator for a few days, then reheated in a pan.

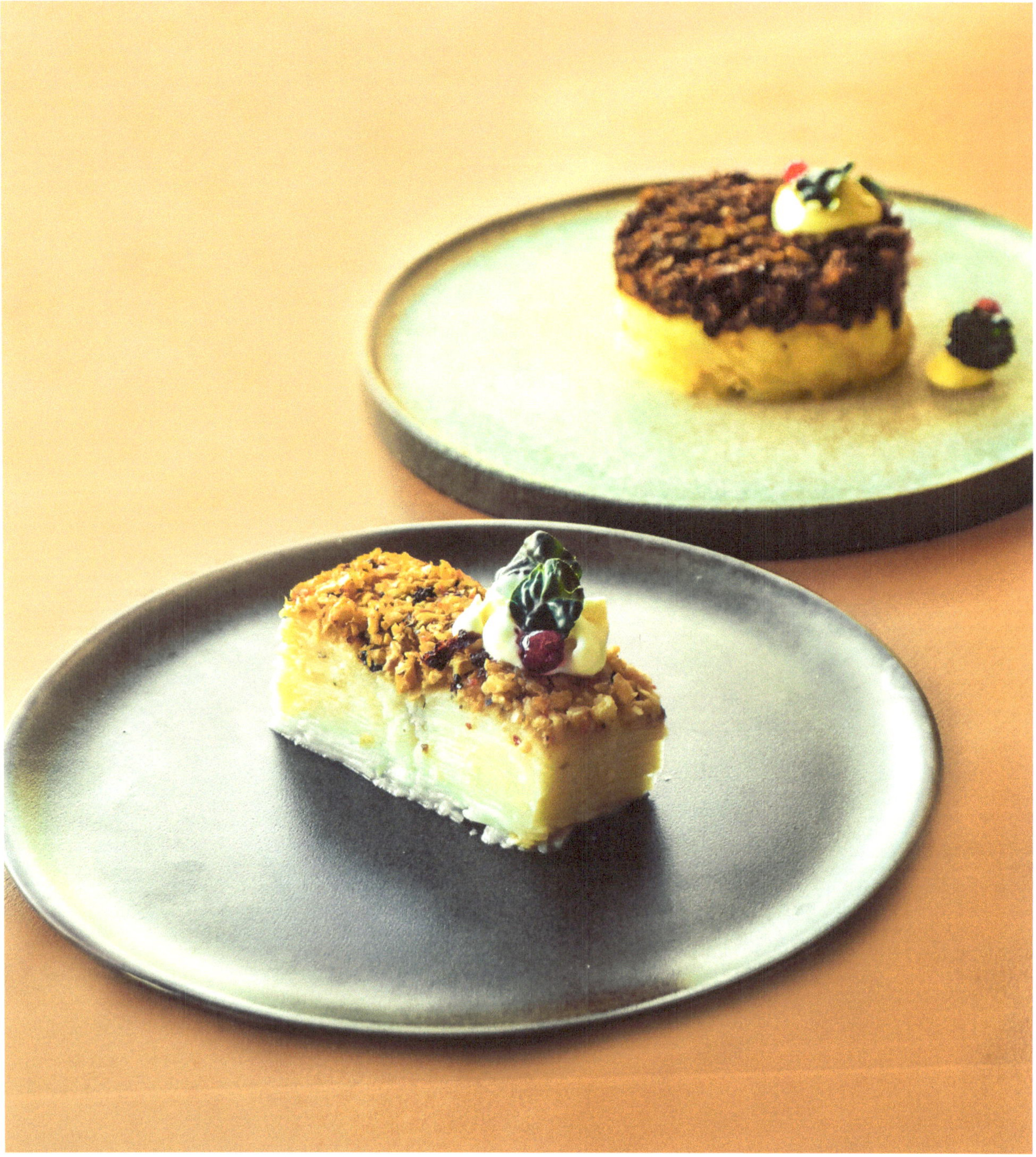

CELERIAC PAVE
WITH ALMOND CREAM AND CELERIAC CRUMB

Time - 20 min. prep + 80 min. cooking
Serves - 6 person

1 kg celeriac
200 ml water
70 g gluten-free rolled oats
Salt to season

To serve
Celeriac crumb (page 23)
Almond cream (page 67)
1 tsp balsamic to serve (optional)

TIPS - Use the kohlrabi, potatoes, beets or other root vegetables in the place of celeriac if you prefer. Follow the same steps for each vegetable. Potatoes may need to cook longer than the celeriac.

Preheat the oven to 180° C.

In a blender, process water, oats and salt together. Place into a mixing bowl.
Peel the celeriac and slice on a mandoline as thin as possible. Line a loaf pan with parchment and place down a layer of the celeriac slices, then brush with oat mixture Repeat this layering until all the celeriac has been used.

Cover the loaf pan with a lid or foil and bake for 1 hour 20 minutes or so, until the celeriac is tender. Allow to cool. Cut a sheet of parchment to lay on top of the terrine in the loaf pan and top with a heavy weight so that the terrine will compact and become stable for slicing.
Refrigerate overnight with the weight on top.

Remove the weights from the Celeriac Pavé, unmould and trim the edges if you prefer. Slice lengthwise into pieces. Place the pieces onto a parchment-lined baking sheet, brush some balsamic and warm gently in the oven for about 20 minutes.

Remove from the oven and top with a generous layer of celeriac crumb. Transfer to plates and top with dollops of cream and balsamic if desired.

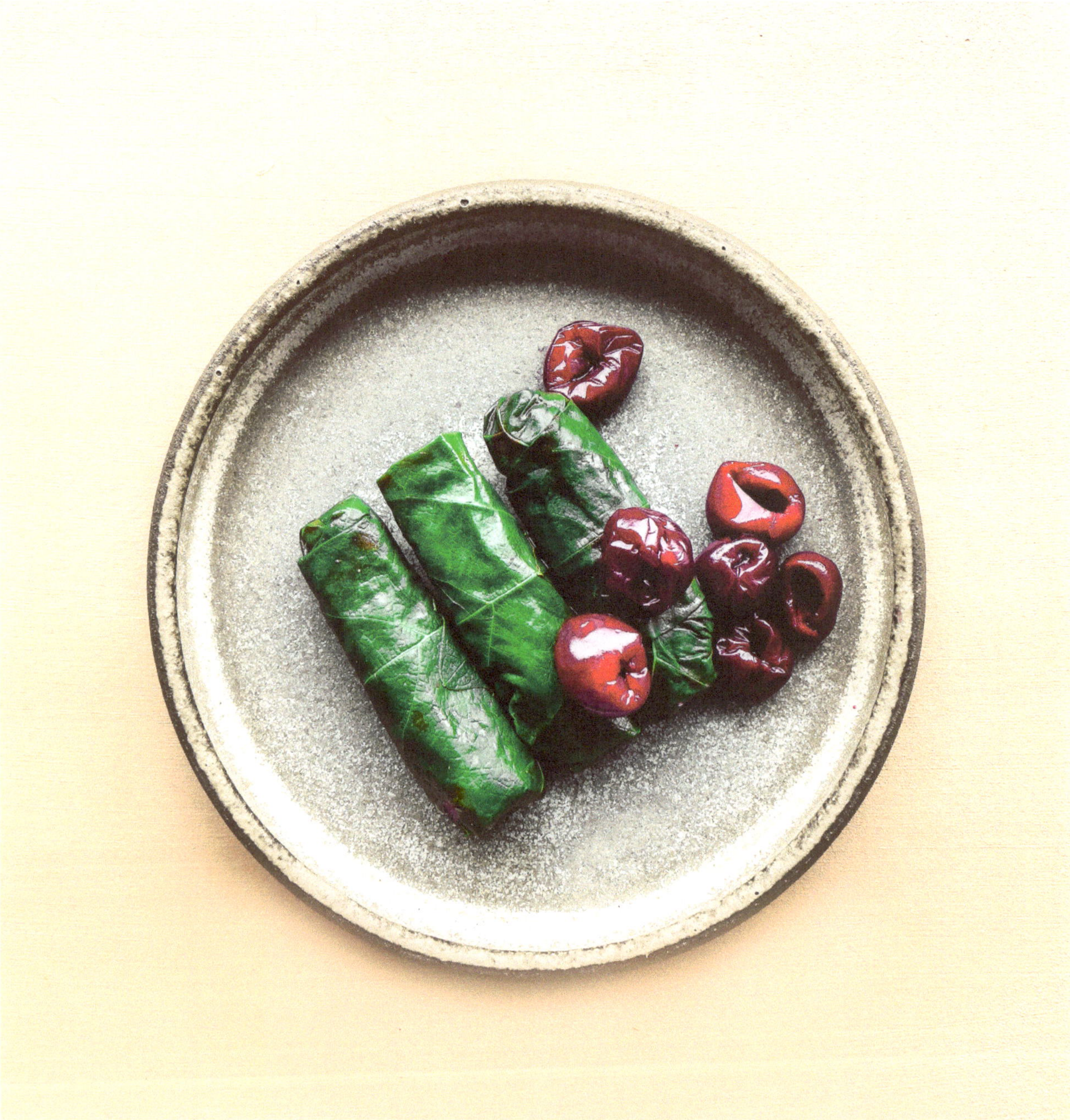

OAT FILLED STUFFED GRAPE LEAVES WITH CHERRIES

Time - 85 minutes

Serves - 6 Servings (about 10 sarmas per serving)

60 fresh grape leaves
4 tbsp cherry juice (from the defrosted cherries)
2 cups hot water
1 cup sour cherries to serve
Lemon wedges to serve
Fresh mint leaves

Filling

60 ml beetroot broth
3 red onions chopped finely
3 garlic cloves minced
1/2 cup sour cherries pitted defrosted
40 g pine nuts
130 g gluten-free rolled oats
1/2 tsp ground cinnamon
1/2 tsp all spice
1/2 tsp dried mint
1 tsp salt

Start by preparing the filling. Soak the oats in slightly warm water for 5 minutes. It shouldn't be too warm or hot, otherwise you will end with a sticky texture and it is hard to handle. Once soaked, strain and remove the excess water.

Meanwhile, heat the beetroot broth in a wide saucepan then add the chopped onions, garlic and pine nuts. Sautee until slightly caramelized. You should still have some beet broth with the caramelized onions, otherwise add extra 2 tbsp beet broth.

Then add the soaked oats into the saucepan and cook for 4-5 minutes or until absorbs the water.

Then add the cinnamon, all spice, dried mint and defrosted pitted cherries. Stir together to combine well. Let the filling cool.

While the filling is cooling off, prepare the vine leaves. If using fresh leaves, put them in hot water for 5 minutes to soften. If using preserved leaves, wash them multiple times to decrease their salt content before putting in hot water.

Oat filled stuffed grape leaves with cherries continued

When the filling is cool enough to handle, you may start assembling. Place each leaf with veins facing up on a level surface, then put a heaping teaspoon of the filling on the bottom half.
Start by folding from the bottom, then fold each side inwards and roll up tightly.

In a wide pan, place a few vine leaves at the bottom to line the surface to prevent the dolmas from burning.
Place all dolmas in the pan, seams facing down, then add the extra cherries, cherry juice from the defrosted cherries and hot water.
Weigh down with a plate and cook, uncovered, for 5 minutes over medium-high heat. Reduce the heat to low, cover the pan, then cook for another 25-30 minutes until they absorb all the water content.

Rest for 10 minutes before serving. It can be served warm or cold. Garnish with cherries and fresh mint leaves if desired.
You may store dolmas in an airtight container for up to five days in the refrigerator. However, they do not freeze very well.

TIPS - Do not cook the rolled oats all the way before assembling, this results in a mushy, offputting texture.
Depending on the depth of your pan, you may need more or less water to cover the surface.
The tartness of the grape leaf is reminiscent of fruit.

Be sure to eat them outdoors, preferably overlooking the sea when it is golden hour.

Have you ever felt a certain joy in dining at golden hours? Any corner of nature can become a great restaurant. First of all, natural light gives back the true colours of the food and normally makes you feel more comfortable than artificial light. Then, in the open air, you can smell the scents more. Moreover, if we have taken a walk to get to the chosen place, even the appetite is felt more strongly.

To experience intense and tasty moments of life, eat in nature!

What is Golden Hour?

Golden hour is the first hour after sunrise and the last hour of light before sunset that produces a warm glowing natural light. That window of time is determined by where you are geographically, as well as the season. Golden hour occurs when the Sun is between six degrees below the horizon and six degrees above.

That's when nature really comes alive. The colours have this soft but deep glow, and all the smells of nature permeate the air.

It feels very special to be out at this time when all the plants and animals start to breathe more deeply. There's a real stillness as the sun goes down. When there's stillness, you can hear very few sounds and see very little movement.

Being in stillness reduces responses in the parasympathetic system, which is responsible for fight or flight and increases responses in the sympathetic system, responsible for rest and relaxation. In other words, it calms your mind allowing you to feel more at peace and less stressed out.

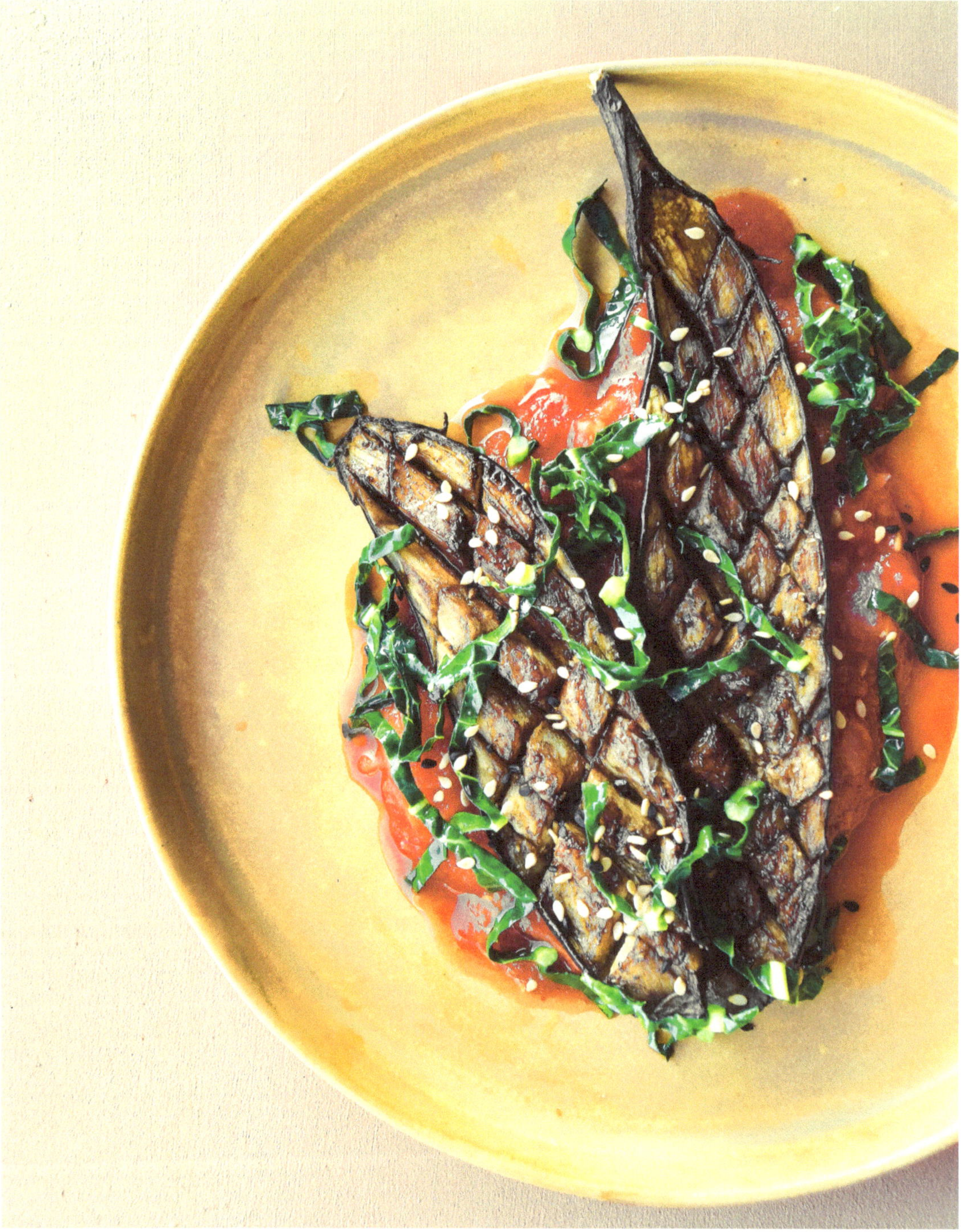

BALSAMIC MUSHROOM GLAZED AUBERGINES WITH GINGER TOMATO SAUCE AND KALE

Time - 50 minutes
Serves - 4 person

2 aubergines split and roasted in halves
4 tbsp beetroot broth + more as needed
Salt to season

Balsamic Mushroom Glaze
1 tbsp minced garlic
100 g sliced mushrooms
30 ml balsamic
50 ml water
A pinch salt and pepper to taste

To Serve
Gingerly tomato sauce (page 37)
Cavolo nero seaweed (page 82)
1 tbsp sesame seeds, lightly toasted

Preheat your oven to 200° C. Cut the aubergines in half, lengthways. Score the flesh in a criss-cross pattern. Drizzle generously with beetroot broth and season with salt. Roast flesh side up for about 30-40 minutes until soft to the core and nicely coloured.

Balsamic Mushroom Glaze
On stove heat garlic on medium high heat for about a minute. Add mushrooms and cook for 3 minutes or until they start to get tender.
Add the balsamic vinegar and let simmer, adding water if need to thin about some. Salt and pepper are added next to taste. Let reduce for about 10 minutes.

Put the roasted aubergine halves flesh side up on a baking sheet and smear with the balsamic mushroom mixture. Grill under a medium grill until the glaze is golden. Scatter with the toasted sesame seeds.

Serve with gingerly tomato sauce and cavolo nero seaweed.

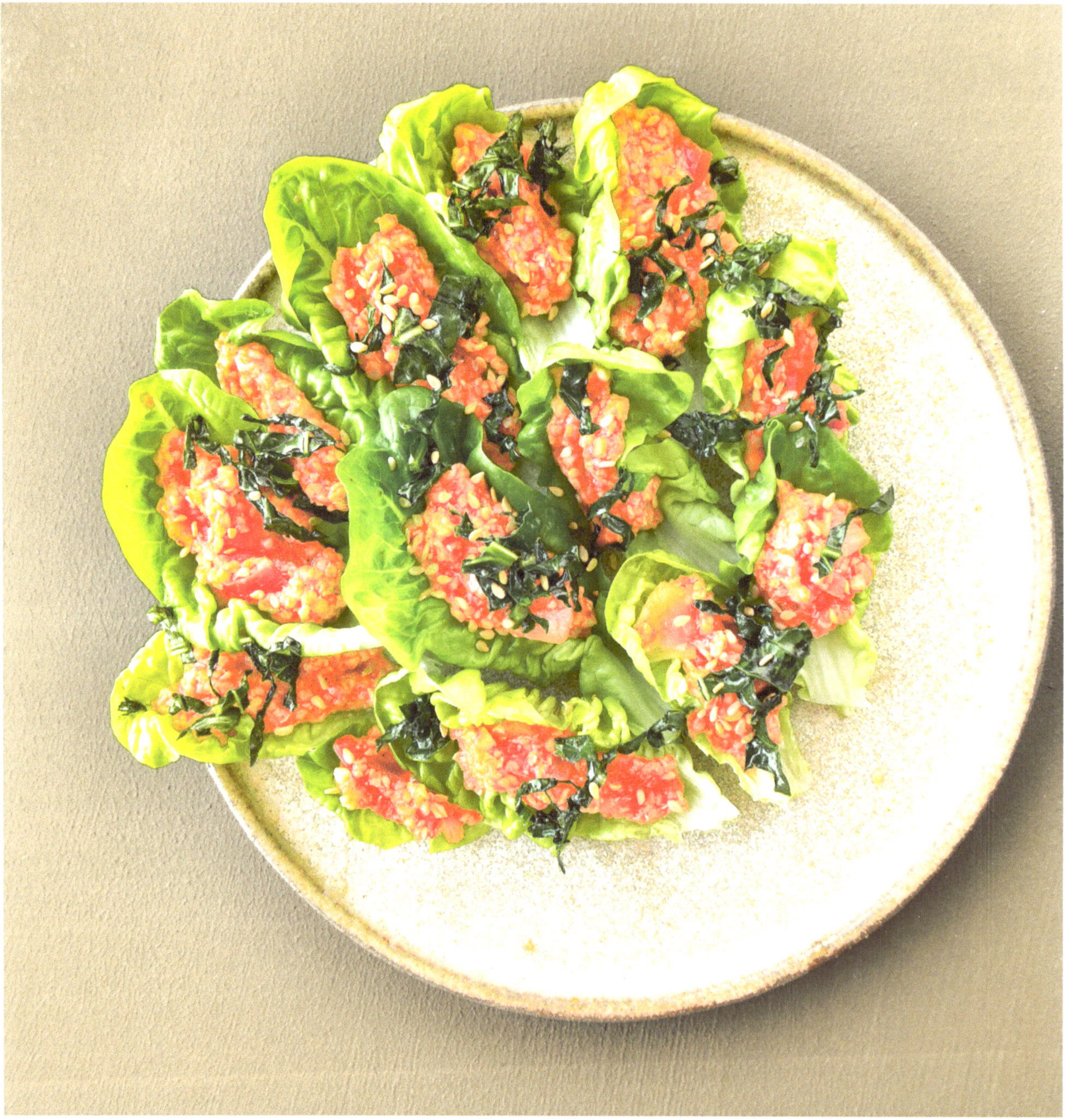

CRACKED BUCKWHEAT FILLED LETTUCE CUPS

These healthy lettuce wraps are filled with tasty combinations of bright sauce, tender cracked buckwheat, and crispy-crunchy cavolo nero. You can also use rolled oats in the place of cracked buckwheat.

Time - 25 minutes
Serves - 6 person

180 g sprouted cracked buckwheat
250 ml water
4 head small lettuce cups
2 tbsp tomato paste
2 large red onion finely chopped
5 garlic cloves minced
1 red bell pepper diced
2 jalapeños diced
60 ml beetroot broth
2 tsp sumac
1 tsp chili flakes
Salt and pepper to taste
Cavolo nero seaweed (page 82)

Place chopped onion, garlic cloves in a large skillet. Add the beet broth and cook for 1-2 minutes until soften, then add the red bell pepper and jalapeños, continue to cook for 2-3 minutes.

Add the tomato paste, 100 ml water, stir until paste.

Add the cracked buckwheat, stir in the paste. Then pour the remaining 150 ml water and cook on low-medium heat until buckwheats absorb the all water content. Taste it, if it is not soften enough, add a little bit more water and continue to cook.

Once cooked, add the sumac and chili flakes. Season with salt and black pepper.

Wash your lettuce cups and drain.

Using a small teaspoon, fill the cups with buckwheat filling. Add the cavolo nero seaweed along with the sesame seeds if desired.

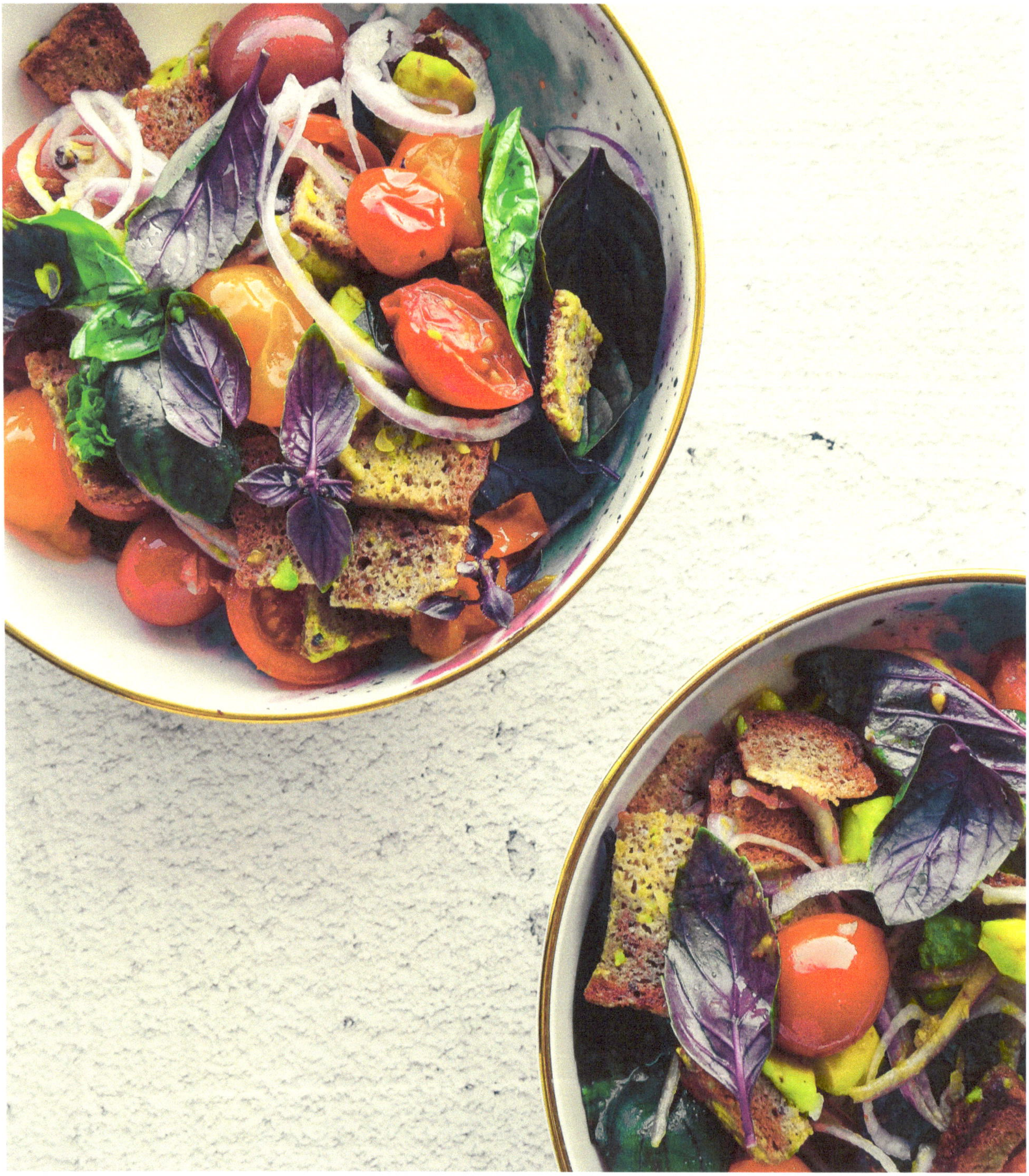

AVOCADO TOMATO PANZANELLA

Panzanella is really a way to use up crusty bread that has gotten hard and to celebrate perfect summer tomatoes. It's best when tomatoes are in season, so make it when you've got super-ripe tomatoes for maximum flavour.

Time - 25 minutes
Serves - 2-3 person

250 g buckwheat loaf of day old bread torn into chunks
500 g mixed cherry tomatoes
2 tbsp balsamic without sugar
1 ripe avocado stoned, peeled and chopped
1 red onion mandolin sliced
2 tbsp pickled caperberries (optional)
1 large clove of garlic crushed
A handful of fresh mixed basil leaves

In a small bowl, mix garlic, balsamic and bread pieces. Toss well to coat everything.
Place in a large non-stick pan and bake on low-medium heat for 15 minutes or until golden brown. Set aside to cool.

Preheat oven to 180º C. In a large oven tray, place the tomatoes, sprinkle with little olive oil and roast until beginning to char. It usually takes 10-15 minutes. Once done, set aside to cool.

In a bowl, mix the thinliy sliced onions with a pinch of salt. Leave to stand for 10 minutes. It will begin to soften quickly.
Place avocados, capers and all the rest into a large salad bowl and sprinkle with the remaining balsamic. Gently mix the salad.

Sprinkle basil leaves and allow to sit for 5-10 minutes before serving.

CAVOLO NERO CRISPY SEAWEED

Time - 20 minutes
Serves - 4

1 large bunch of cavolo nero
2 tbsp lemon juice
2 tbsp sesame seeds
Good pinch of salt
1/4 tsp chili

Toppings
Poppy seeds or sesame of your choice

Preheat oven to 160° C.
Remove the stalks from the kale, then roll up the leaves and finely slice them, so you have thin shreds of kale.

In a mixing bowl, mix the shredded leaves with salt and lemon juice, mixing well to ensure the leaves are coated.

Arrange on a baking tray lined parchment paper, spreading the leaves out evenly so they can crisp up in the oven.

Roast for between 8-10 minutes, checking often and mixing to turn the leaves.

Meanwhile, toast some sesame seeds in a dry frying pan. Stir continuously to stop them catching. Remove from the heat when done.
When the kale is crispy all over, it's done. Sprinkle with the toasted sesame seeds and serve.

This is a quick and tasty approach to cavolo nero and tastes just like the crispy seaweed!

LEEKS WITH POIREAUX VINAIGRETTE

Time - 30 minutes
Serves - 4

500g leeks
1/2 tsp salt
1 pot water to boil

Poireaux Vinaigrette
1 tbsp red wine vinegar or balsamic
5 tbsp white vegetable broth
1 small red onion peeled and finely diced
1 tbsp dijon mustard
2 tbsp chopped parsley
2 tbsp chopped chives
1/2 tsp salt
1/8 tsp black pepper

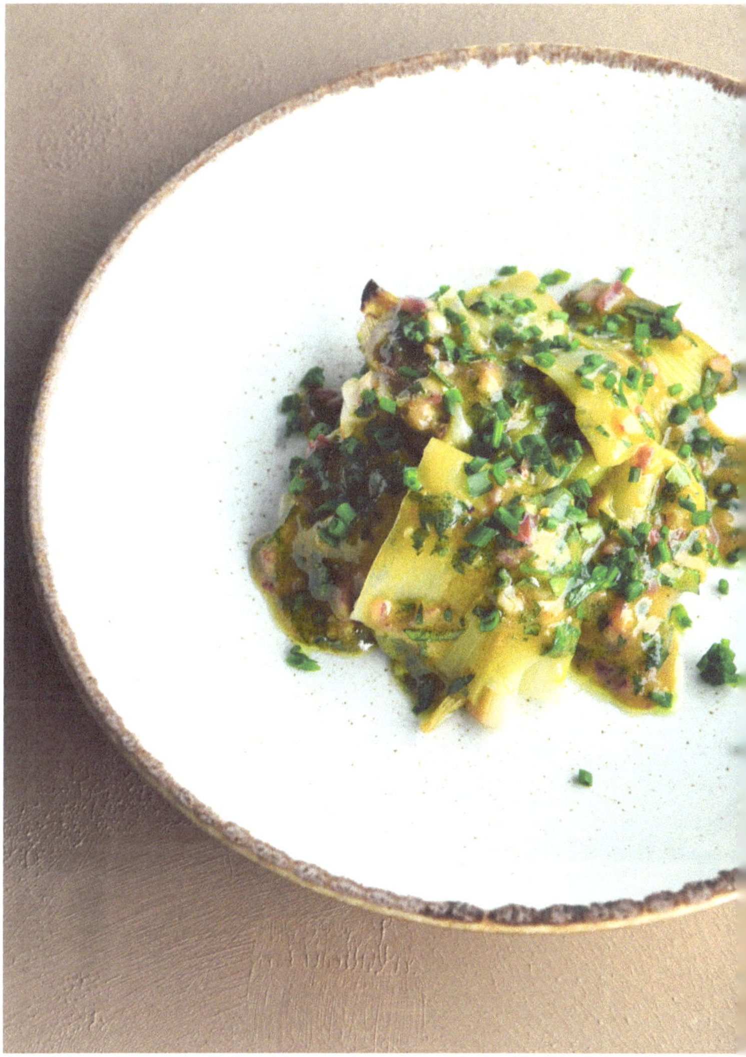

Cut off and discard the root ends of the leeks.
Wash and place in a pot. Cover with water and sprinkle some salt. Cook on medium heat for 20 minutes until the leeks are fork-tender.
To prepare the vinaigrette. Combine the vinegar and salt in a bowl, and whisk with a fork for about 20 seconds until the salt has dissolved. Then add the onion, mustard, parsley, and pepper. Then, slowly drizzle in the vegetable broth in a steady stream while constantly whisking. Continue whisking until the dressing thickens to your desired texture.
Remove the leek bundles from the water with a slotted spoon and let them cool and drain on a kitchen towel.

Using your hands, roll or fold the leeks. Dip in the sauce.
Place the leeks on a serving platter, sprinkle some chives.

Top generously with the vinaigrette. Serve warm or at room temperature.

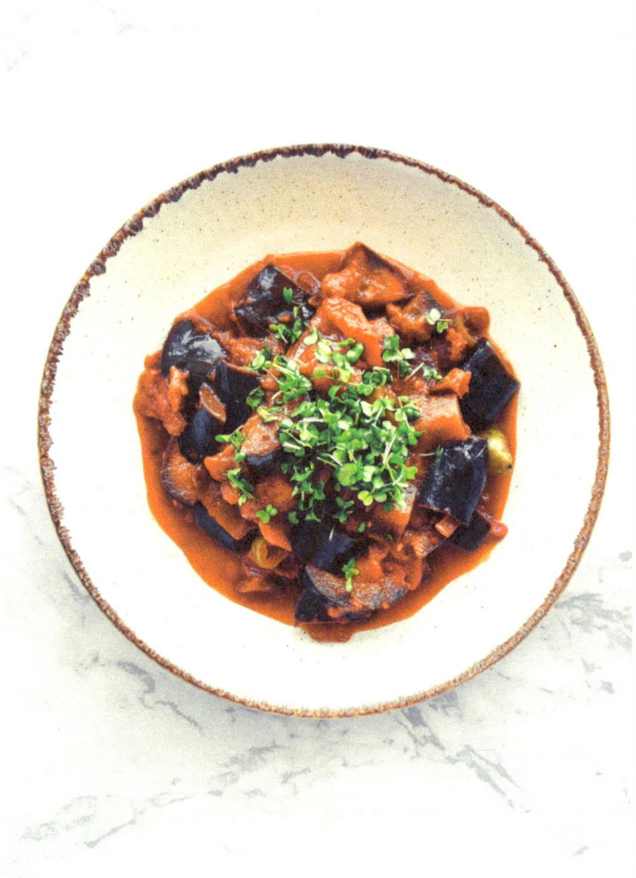

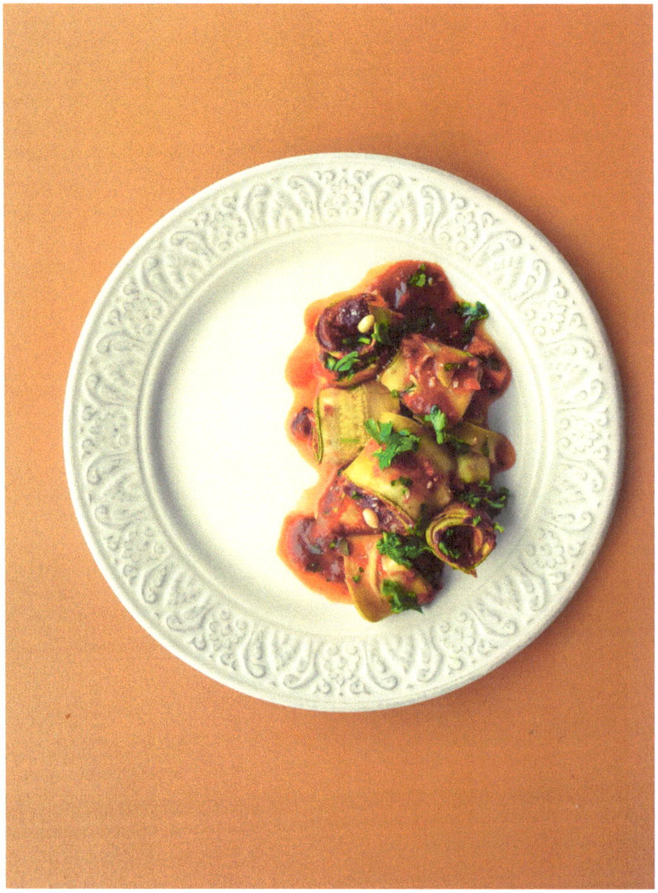

EGGPLANT STEW WITH SUGAR PLUMS AND JALAPENO

Time - 30 minutes
Serves - 4

4 large eggplants cubed
1 ripe sugar plum
3 small fresh jalapeño
1 garlic clove minced
3 large tomatoes chopped
1 tbsp tomato paste
1 red onion chopped
1/2 tsp salt or more if you need
2 tbsp beetroot broth
150 to 200 ml water
Pepper to taste
Microgreens to serve

In a large pot, add the chopped tomatoes, plums, jalapeños, garlic, salt and beet broth. Cook on medium heat until soften. Then add the tomato paste and stir. Cook until thick enough. Then set aside.

In a separate pot, cook the chopped onions with a little bit beet broth until soften. Then add cubed eggplants into the pot. Toss together. Cook for 2-3 minutes stirring occasionally. Then add some water, close the lif of the pot, cook on medium heat for 15 minutes or until soften.

Once soften, add the tomato plum sauce, stir well.

Continue to cook until eggplants are soften enough and absorb the water. Serve with micro greens, pepper and salt.

ZUCCHINI INVOLTINI WITH MUSHROOM BOLOGNESE

Time - 40 minutes
Serves - 4

3-4 large zucchini
2 medium red onion finely chopped
3 garlic cloves minced
1 medium carrot diced
2 tbsp mushroom stock (or tamari, coconut aminos)
1/4 cup beet stock (page 28)
1 large red bell pepper diced
1 tsp chili flakes
200 g finely chopped mushrooms
2 tbsp tomato paste
1/4 bunch fresh parsley or basil to serve
Sunflower hemp crumble to serve (page 23)
Salt and pepper to taste

Preheat oven to 200° C.

To make filling, in a large skillet, saute the onions, garlic, carrot, red bell pepper and mushrooms together along with the mushroom stock in the beet stock until transculent. Trim the stem end of each zucchini. Stand each vertically, and make ¼-inch thick cuts down to create long slices. Season with salt and pepper. Meanwhile, mix the tomato paste with some water to thin, season with salt and chili. Place a spoonful of filling at one end of each of the zucchini slices. Roll the slice into a tight coil and place it seam-side down in the pan on top of the tomato sauce. Bake for 20 minutes.

Serve with chopped parsley and nut crumble.

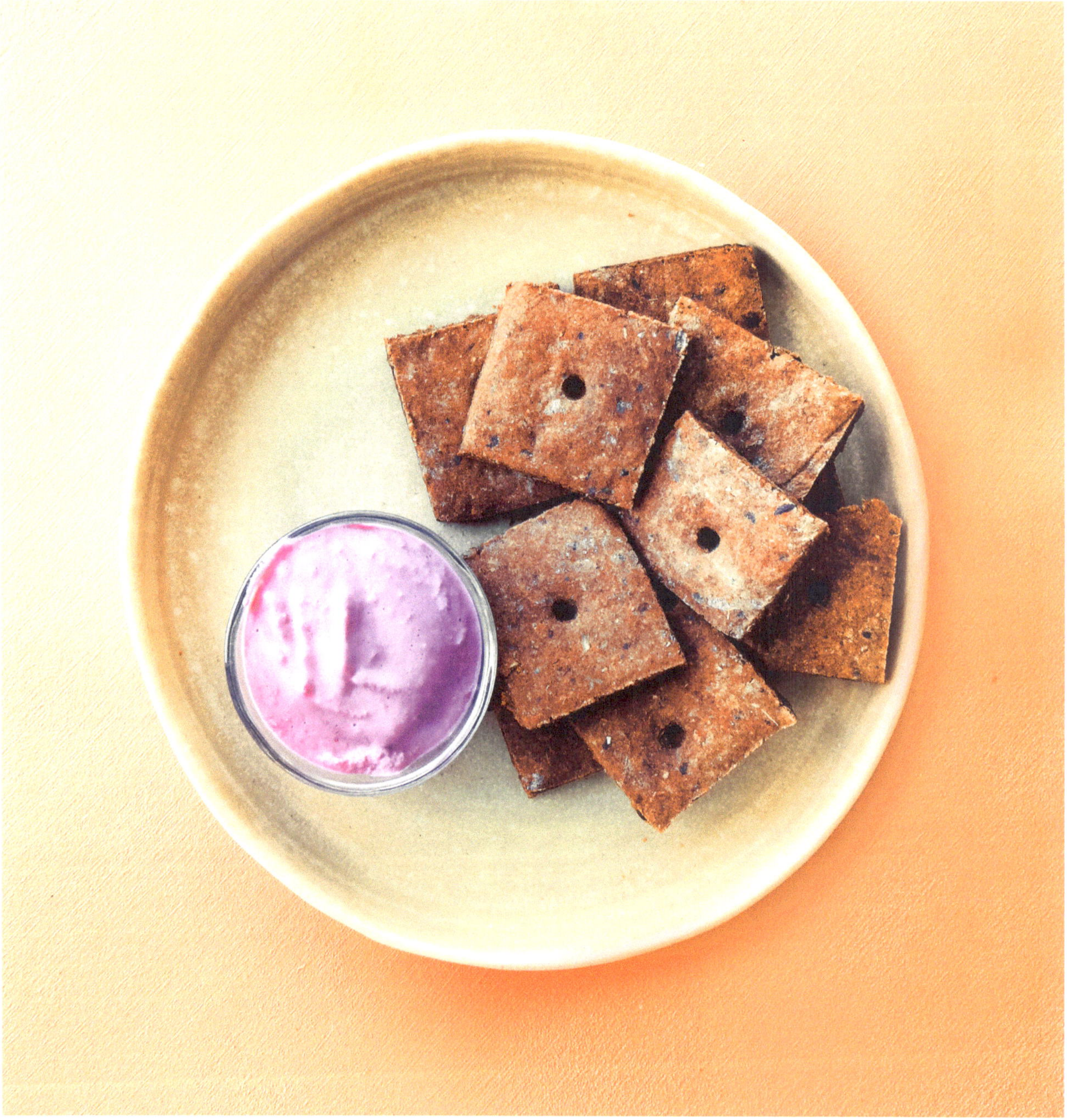

TEFF PIZZA CRACKERS

All the flavors of pizza in the cracker form! These crackers are great to add to a dip platter or enjoy as it is. Also can be used as a pizza crust, top with your favorite toppings.

Time - 15 min prep + 20 min baking
Serves - 25 crackers cut into 2x2 squares

Wet Ingredients

1 tbsp flaxseed + 3 tbsp water
15 g sunflower seed butter
2 tsp apple cider vinegar
1 large soft date mashed or 1 tsp grape molasses
4 tbsp plant milk
35 g tomato paste
2 garlic cloves minced
4-5 large leaves of fresh basil chopped finely

Dry Ingredients

55 g teff flour
50 g gluten-free oat flour
35 g brown rice flour
1/2 tsp dried oregano
1/2 tsp red pepper flakes
1/2 tsp salt
1/2 tsp baking soda
1 tsp onion powder or asafoetida
1 tsp italian blend of herbs

Preheat oven to 190° C.

In a medium bowl, whisk together all the dry ingredients. Set aside.

Grind your flaxseed in a coffee grinder. Make the flax egg by mixing the ground flaxseed with the cold water. Let stand for 5 minutes to thicken.

In a small bowl whisk together the remaining wet ingredients.

Add the dry ingredients and flax mixture into wet mixture and mix until dough comes together into a ball.

Let the dough rest in the refrigerator for 5 minutes.

Place a piece of parchment on your workspace, cutting a second piece the same size to sandwich the dough between to prevent sticking. Begin by flattening the dough with your hands on the parchment paper. If it is too sticky, sprinkle with a little teff flour. It may crack a little at the sides when you are pushing it out, but just mold this back into shape with your hands.

Once it is less than an inch thick, place the second piece of parchment on top and begin evenly rolling the dough out with a rolling pin. Once you have rolled it out to about 3mm thick you can remove the top piece of parchment and score the cracker into squares. Slide the crackers on the parchment onto a large sheet tray. Bake in the oven for 18- 20 minutes, or until golden and crisp. Watch carefully at the 15-minute mark as the crackers can burn easily and you may need to remove the edge crackers first if they are thinner and have cooked faster. Allow to cool and enjoy with dips!

SIMPLE DOESN'T ALWAYS MEAN QUICK OR SHORT RECIPES, IT REQUIRES UNDERSTANDING WHY WE DO HOW WE DO.

GLUTEN-FREE FLOUR MIX

This chapter is devoted to healthy versions of my classic favorites. Even tough there is no one right way of doing healthy, I believe making from strach with minimally processed ingredients is the best possible way.

In the dough based recipes, I usually simply use a base recipe that I've developed and there may be changes in the ratio according to the recipe.

The main ingredient is buckwheat flour (sprouted or regular one, both will work.) , and as a starch I always add half amount of the buckwheat flour I put in, I prefer cassava as the healthiest and less processed ingredient (alternatively arrowroot or tapioca can be used). Cassava or tapioca gives softness to the dough, while psyllium provides flexibility.

You can reduce buckwheat flour by 25% and add alternatives such as oat flour, teff flour, sorghum flour, brown rice flour, amaranth flour,chickpea flour or quinoa flour. If you want to remove the starch from the dough, you will get a tough texture and crumbly buckwheat dough. Even if you add psyllium, it will be difficult to work with the dough as it will not give enough softness.

When you learn this simple information, you can easily develop new combinations with different flours by following this base recipe. (page 117)

If your dough is tough, you can proceed by adding a little more water, or if it is sticky, you can add a little more flour.

USING BEETROOT STOCK INSTEAD OF OIL

Instead of oil, I often use beet stock which was my life-saving invention last year. Especially when sautéing the onions in the pan, they get caramelized wonderfully in the beetroot stock and soften nicely.

A mixture of beet juice and balsamic (without sugar) is also a good alternative. In general, I use both together, the ratio is 1:1.

White and brown vegetable stock recipes are given at the beginning of the book. You can also use the appropriate one according to the type of food you are going to make.

I will usually be using beet stock (page 25) for sautéing. This book is a guide to encourage and show you new ways to cook without oil. But if oil is not an issue for you, you can use the oil of your choice for the parts where the beet broth is used for sautéing, baking or frying.

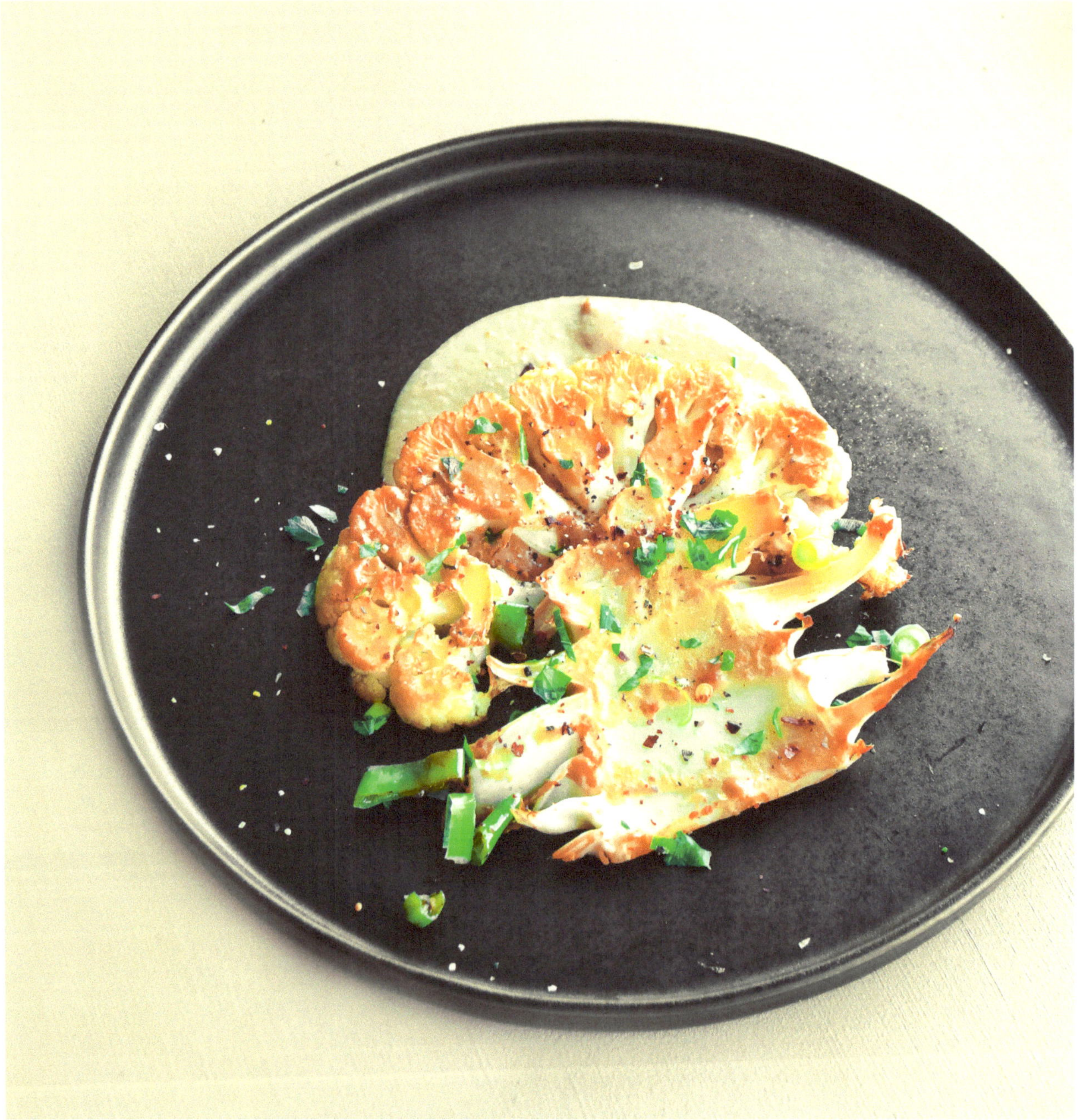

CAULIFLOWER STEAK WITH THAI SAUCE

Making cauliflower steak is actually very easy. Slice, season, and roast in a hot oven! It's one of the easiest cauliflower recipes and very satisfying!

Time - 20 min prep + 30 min cooking
Serves - 1 big batch

200 ml vegetable broth mixed with 1/2 tsp salt
1 large head cauliflower sliced into steaks
2 thinly sliced jalapeños to serve
2 springs green onions to serve
1/4 cup finely chopped parsley

Thai Peanut Sauce
1 small red onion minced
3 garlic cloves minced
1 tbsp galangal or fresh ginger grated
60 g peanut butter unsweetened
2 tamarind pitted or sukkari dates
90-120 ml water as needed to thin
2 tbsp mushroom stock (page 30, or use reduced sodium tamari or coconut aminos)
1 tbsp maple syrup (or grape molasses)
1 tsp chili
1/4 tsp salt

TIPS

If you have peanut allergy, use other kind of nuts like almond butter. For those who have nut allergy use sunflower seed butter or simply replace with tomato sauce.

Preheat oven to 250° C. Remove the leaves of the cauliflower and trim the end of stems leaving core intact. The stem is needed to keep the 'steaks' intact. Place cauliflower core side down on a work surface. Using a large knife, slice cauliflower into four 1/2" steaks from center of cauliflower (some florets will break loose; bake them too).
Heat 60 ml of vegetable broth in a large heavy ovenproof skillet over medium-high heat. Working in 3-4 batches, cook cauliflower steaks until golden brown and fork tender, about 2 minutes per side, adding another 60 ml broth (or more as needed) to pan between batches. Transfer steaks to a large rimmed baking sheet.

In the meantime, make your peanut sauce, add all ingredients from red onion to chili to a food processor or blender and blend until smooth. Brush the top side of the steaks with the peanut sauce, reserving half for later. Place the tray in the oven and roast for 15 minutes until just tender and the edges are charring. Carefully turn the steaks and brush with the half of the remaining mixture. Roast for a further 15 - 20 minutes. Pour the rest of the sauce in the plate. Plate up and sprinkle with the chopped parsley, green onions, jalapeño and the remaining sauce. Sprinkle some salt.
To make it a full meal, include a side of whole grains like brown basmati rice, quinoa or buckwheat and greens, like organic kale, chard, or spinach.

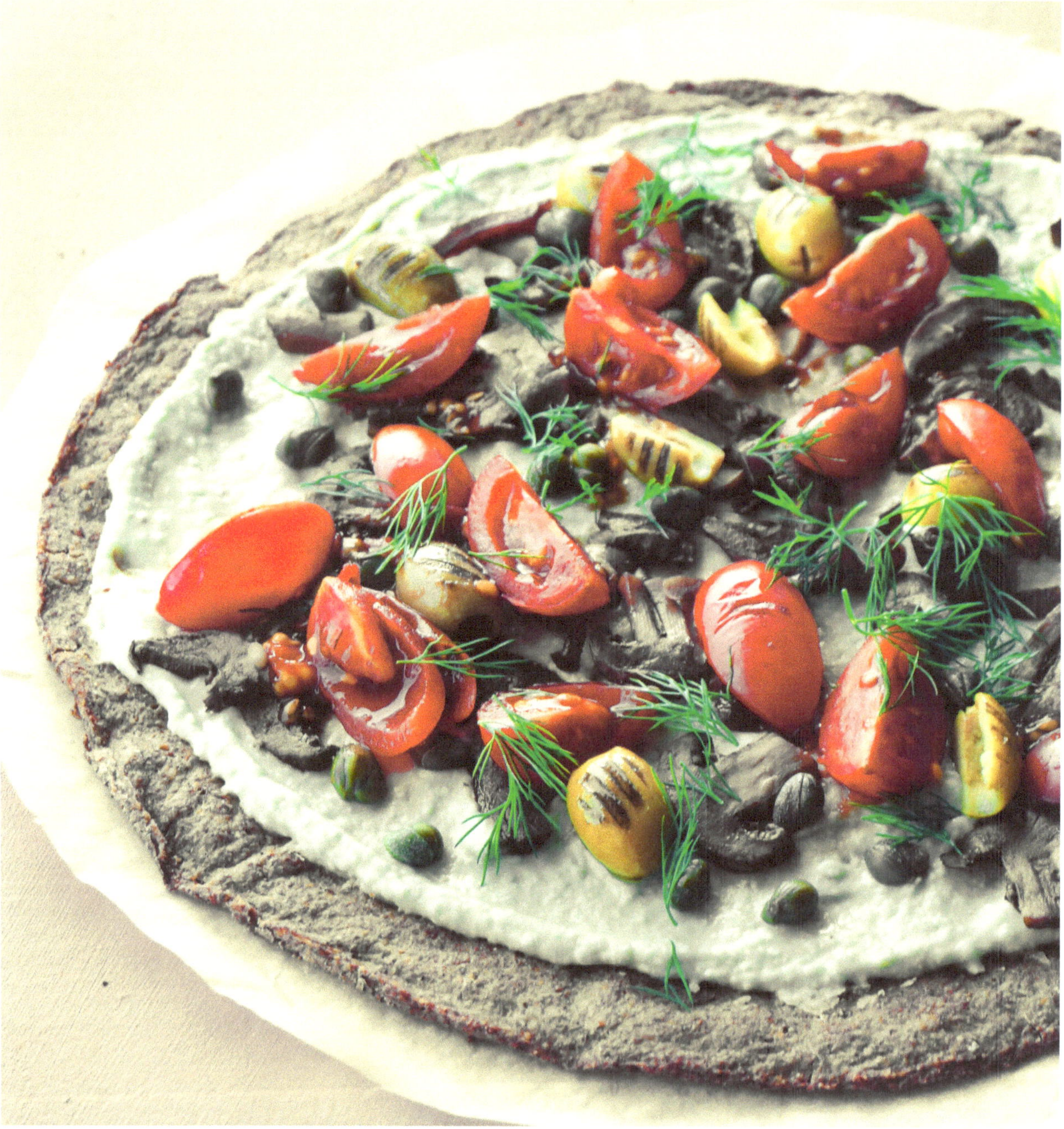

CAULIFLOWER PIZZA

Time - 45 minutes
Yield - 30 cm pizza

400 g cauliflower florets
30 g chia seeds + 175 ml water
80 g almond flour (or chickpea flour)
1/2 tsp garlic powder
1/2 tsp salt

Toppings
Bean cream (page 34)
Caperberries
Olives
Fresh dill chopped
Sauted mushrooms
Cherry tomatoes quartered

Preheat oven to 200° C, line a large baking sheet with parchment paper.

Fill a large pot with an inch of water, then place a steamer basket over that. Fill the basket with the fresh cauliflower florets and bring the water to a boil. Once boiling, cover the pot and lower the heat to a simmer. Cook until the cauliflower is very tender, about 10 to 15 minutes. Drain and transfer the cauliflower to a food processor. Process it briefly to make cauliflower rice.

Transfer the cooked cauliflower rice to a strainer. Using the back of a spoon, press down, removing all of the excess moisture.

In a small bowl, mix the chia and water together. Let it sit for 15 minutes.

In a large bowl mix the garlic, salt and almond flour together. Then add the chia mixture and cauliflower rice. Stir well to combine together.

Press the mixture into the parchment-lined baking sheet, using your hands or a spatula to shape the crust into your desired size. The thinner and flatter you can press the crust, the better, but try to keep it as even as possible for a sturdy result.

Bake the crust at 200° C for 25 minutes, checking on it after 30 minutes to make sure it's not starting to burn. You want the crust to be dry to the touch and lightly browned with crispy edges.

Once the crust is firm and dry, add your favorite pizza toppings and return to the oven briefly to let everything heat up, about 5-10 additional minutes. Serve warm.

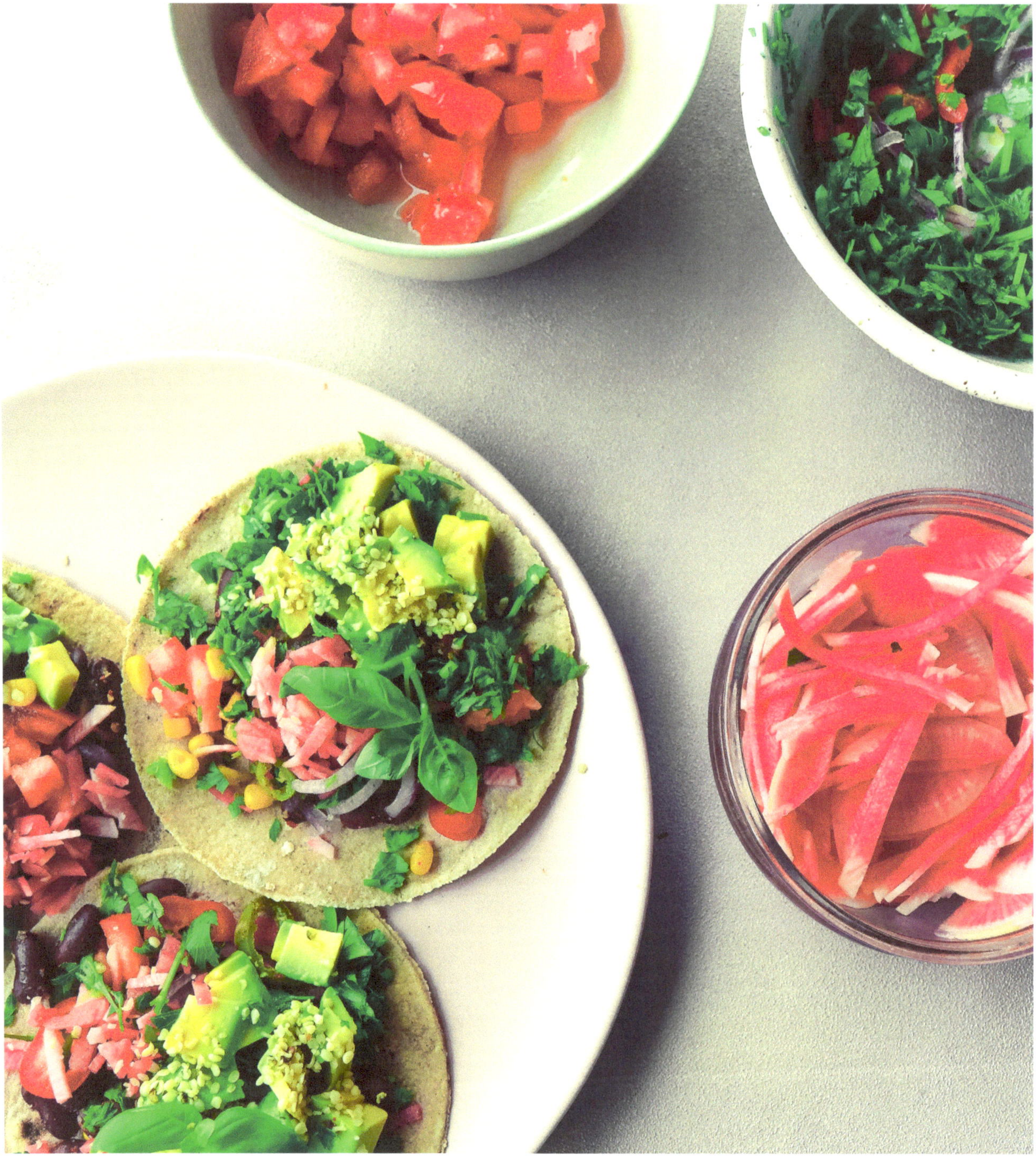

BUCKWHEAT RAINBOW TACOS

The toasted-seed nuttiness of rustic, toothsome buckwheat tortillas mellows with lemon-fresh avocado, radish, mexican beans, corns and hot jalapeños. So delicious and easy to make!

Time - 30 minutes
Serves -4 person

Dough

120 g (1 cup) buckwheat flour
65 g (1/2 cup) cassava or tapioca flour
1 tbsp psyllium powder + 3 tbsp water
1/4 tsp salt
90 ml water

Filling

1/2 cup thinly sliced discs of watermelon radish tossed with 1 tbsp apple cider vinegar
1/2 bunch chopped fresh basil (or cilantro, parsley)
1 small red onion finely chopped
2-3 thinly sliced jalapeños
1 ripe avocado cut into small pieces
200 g cooked mexican beans
100 g cooked corn
100 g diced tomatoes
Salt and red pepper to season
Hemp hearts to top (optional)

In a large mixing bowl, mix the psyllium with 3 tbsp water, stir well. Then add the buckwheat flour, tapioca, salt and rest of the water. Mix well until you get dough form.
Remove dough from the bowl, knead with your hands. Dust some buckwheat flour on your work surface. Roll the dough thinly as much as possible but avoiding the breaking.

Using a 7-8 cm round cutter, cut your dough into small tortillas. Heat a non-stick pan on medium-high heat. Put a tortilla in the pan. Bake both sides for 1-2 minutes monitoring carefully in order to avoid burning. Repeat the process for the rest.

Using a mandoline slicer, thinly slice your radish then cut into matchsticks using a chef knife. Place in a bowl, toss with apple cider vinegar. Let it sit for 5 minutes.

In a pan, add the beetroot broth, chopped red onion, jalapeños and red bell pepper. Saute for 2-3 minutes until soften. Then add the cooked mexican beans and corn continue to cook for about 3-4 minutes. Add some salt and red pepper flakes.
Serve tortillas with bean corn mixture, marinated radish matchsticks, diced avocados, tomatoes and fresh basil, chopped parsley or cilantro. Add some extra red onion finely sliced if you like. Sprinkle some hemp hearts on top if desired.

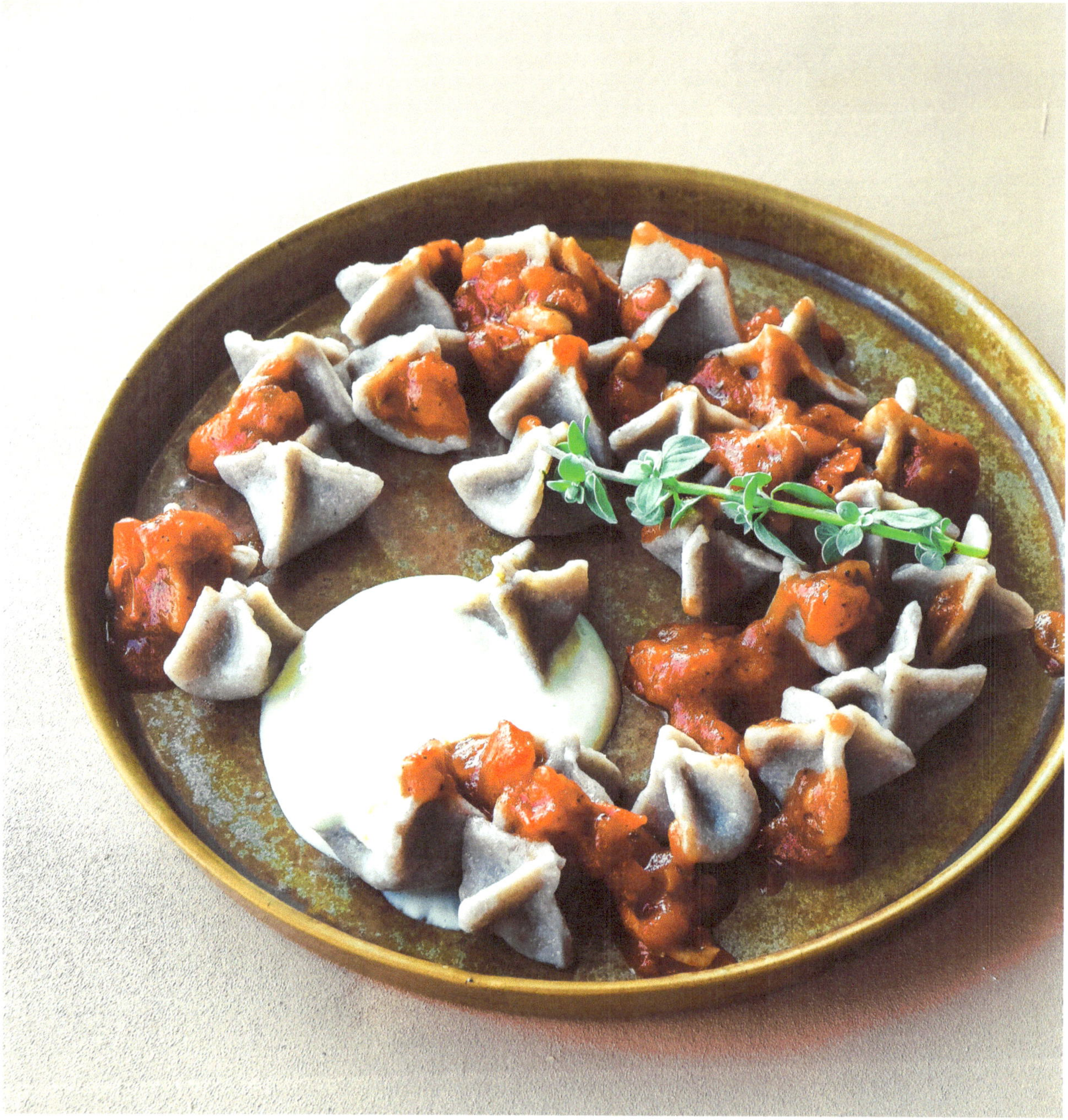

SPINACH DUMPLINGS WITH TOMATO SAUCE AND YOGURT

Time - 1 hour

Serves - 2 person

Dough

120 g sprouted buckwheat flour
65 g cassava or tapioca flour
1 tbsp psyllium husk powder
125 ml filtered water
1/2 tsp salt

Spinach Filling

400 g fresh spinach
1 large onion chopped
Black pepper and salt to taste

Tomato Sauce

400 g chopped tomatoes
2 garlic cloves minced
1 tsp sumac
1 tsp salt
2-3 tbsp water as needed
1 tbsp chopped fresh rosemary
(or fresh majoram)

Yogurt

150g silken tofu (oat, soy or
hemp tofu of your choice)
1-2 tbsp water as needed
2 garlic cloves minced
3 tbsp lemon juice
1/2 tsp salt

To make spinach filling, chop your onion and place in a pan, add 2-3 tbsp water to saute. Once onions are soften, chop the washed, drained spinach leaves. Then add to the pan, toss with the onions, cook for 2-3 minutes on medium heat. Once they become bright green, strain the excess water and remove. Set aside to cool down.

To make the dough, place the buckwheat flour, cassava flour, psyllium husk and salt in a large mixing bowl. Stir to combine well. Then add the water, immediately mix with a spoon until everything combined well. Start kneading with your hands. The dough should be a bit fluffy, elastic and smooth. Once done, Take out of the mixing bowl.
Sprinkle some buckwheat flour on your work surface. Place the dough. Using a rolling pin, roll the dough out about 0.5 mm thick. Cut into 1x1 cm squares.
Place a tiny amount of filling inside each square and fold from the corners.
Drop them in salted boiling water and cook until they rise on the surface of the water.

For the sauce, crush the garlic cloves and mix them silken tofu in the blender. Add the lemon juice, salt and 1-2 tbsp water as needed. Refrigerate for a thick consistency.
In a sauce pan, cook the garlic and tomatoes together until soften. Add 1-2 tbsp pasta water to get a nice smooth tomato sauce. Once done, add the rosemary, sumac and salt.
Serve your dumplings with yogurt and tomato sauce, adjust the salt and herbs.

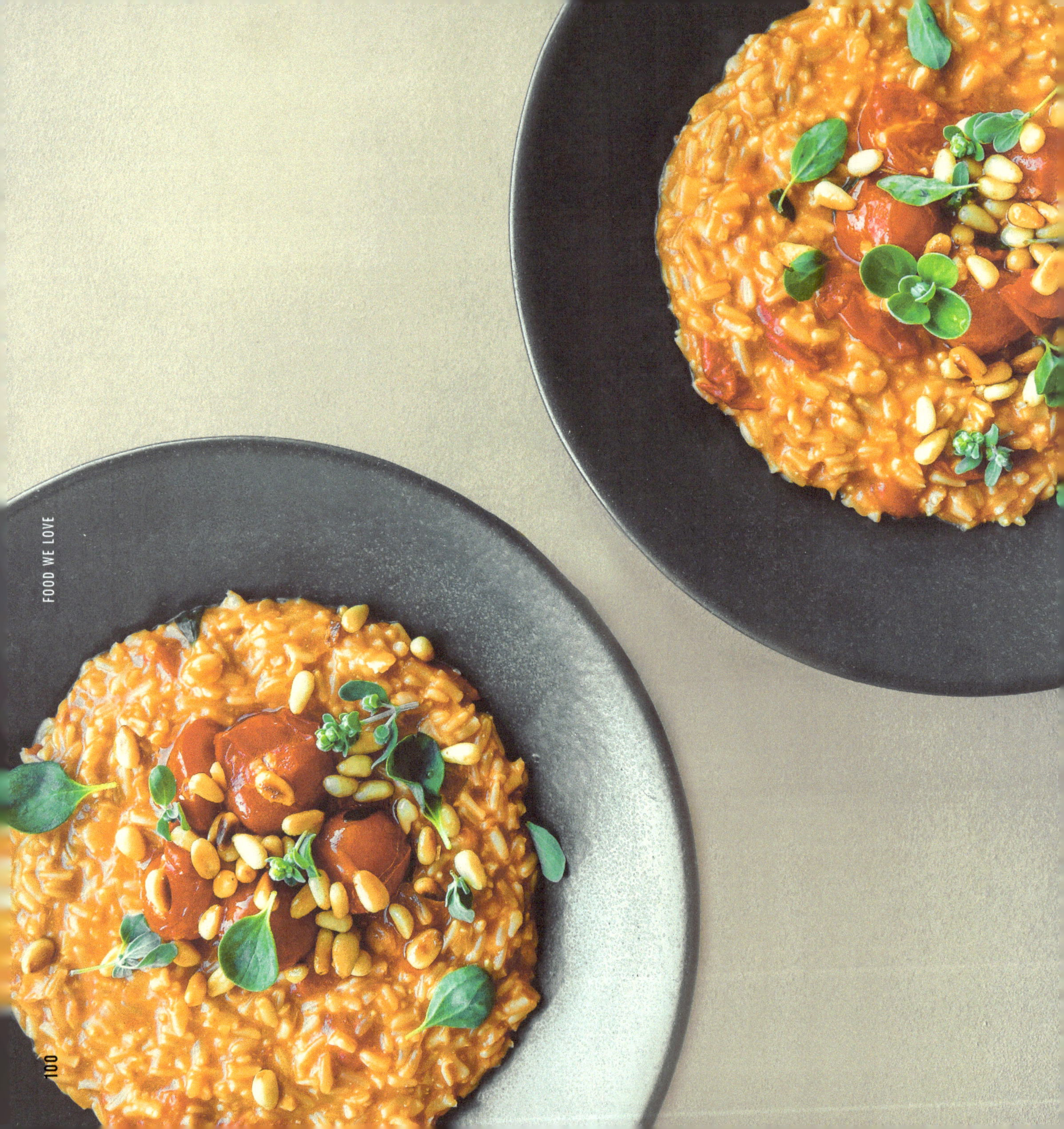

WHOLE OAT RISOTTO WITH PLUM AND TOMATOES

Oats release a lot of starch as they cook, which is exactly what makes risotto so great, and if you follow the same procedure of making regular risotto and stirring constantly, you will end up with something of a similar texture as risotto.

Time - 40 minutes
Serves - 2 person

500g ripe tomatoes
1 ripe plum
150g whole oats
1 cup filtered water
3 garlic cloves minced

Add-Ons
1 tsp salt
1/2 tsp seaweed blend (optional)
Freshly grounded blackpepper
Sunflower hemp crumb to serve (page 23)
Toasted pine nuts to serve
Herbs of your choice (majoram, rosemary or basil. Use only one.)

Place whole oats in a bowl, wash and dry. Cover with water, let it sit overnight or for 10-12 hours.
Then strain the excess water. Set aside.

Wash and cut your tomatoes and plums, place in a deep pot, add the minced garlic.

Cook on medium-low heat for 15-20 minutes or until tomatoes leave their juice and they are soft enough. Then add the whole oats, cook another 20 minutes until oats absorbs the water.

Add 1/2 cup to 1 cup filtered water as needed depending on water content in the tomatoes you might need to add more water. Taste it if it is too thick, add more water and continue to cook. It should be a bit juicy, not too thick. Once cooked, let it sit for 8-10 minutes before serving.

Season with salt, seaweed and black pepper. Serve with sunflower hemp crumb or plant-based nut parmesan, toasted pine nuts and herbs of your choice.

TIPS - If you can't find the whole oats, you can also use steel-cut oats, risotto rice or other types of rice you prefer.

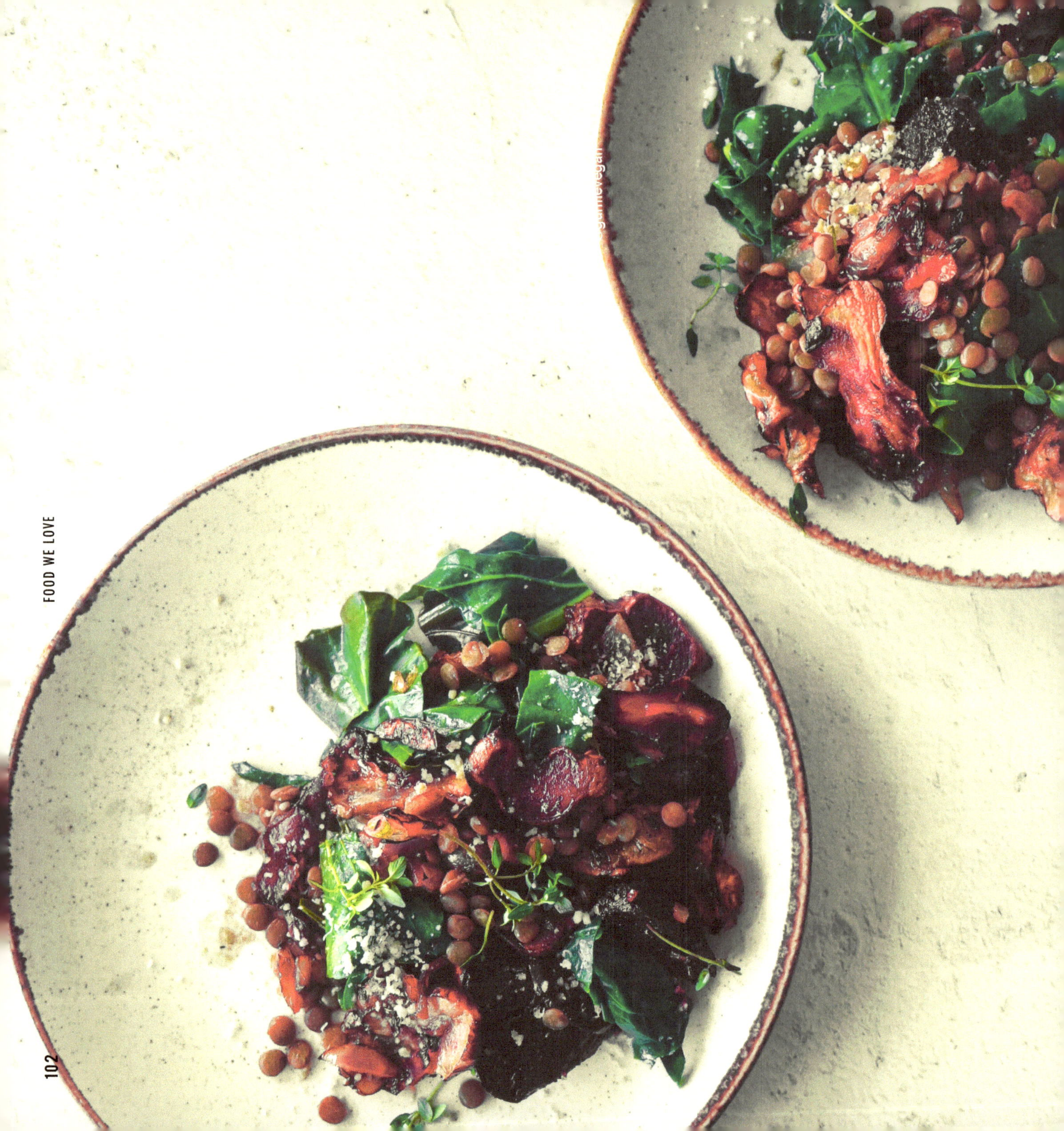

GREEN LENTILS WITH BEETS SUNCHOKES AND SWISS CHARD

Time - 45 minutes
Serves - 4 person

3-4 small beets
7-8 large chard
250 g sunchokes
3 tbsp balsamic
4 tbsp beet broth
200 g cooked green lentil
1 large red onion diced

2 garlic cloves minced
1-2 tbsp balsamic vinegar
4-5 tbsp sunflower hemp crumb to serve (page 23)
Fresh thyme
Salt and blackpepper to taste

Preheat oven to 200° C.
Scrub and trim beets and sunchokes and cut into ½ inch slices or wedges. Place on a foil lined baking sheet. Drizzle 1 tbsp balsamic and 2 tbsp beetroot broth and roast until tender, about 30 minutes.
To cook lentils, place green lentils in a small pot and cover with 3 inches of water and a pinch salt. Bring to a boil, cover and turn heat down to a simmer, cook until tender (it usually takes 20 minutes, should still hold their shape.) Then Drain.
In a large skillet, heat the remaining 2 tablespoons beet broth over medium high heat. Add diced onion and saute 3-4 minutes. Turn heat down to medium, add garlic and cook 2 more minutes, until golden and fragrant. Add more beet broth or water if necessary.
Lower heat to medium low. Add chard and gently wilt, just slightly, about 2-3 more minutes. Season with salt and pepper.
Add cooked lentils to the skillet, gently folding them in and warming.
Add beets and sunchokes then splash with 1-2 tablespoons balsamic vinegar. Let vinegar cook down for just a couple minutes so it's not so acidic. Sprinkle with nut parmesan and fresh thyme if you like.
Taste again, if it tastes bland it most likely needs salt. Serve immediately.

PASTA WITH BEETROOT SAUCE

Time - 1 hour
Serves - 2-3 person

250 g gluten-free pasta of your choice (I used yellow pea pasta)
200 g beetroot
1/4 cup (60 ml) beet broth
1 tbsp lemon juice or vinegar
1 cup (240 ml) almond milk
1 red onion chopped
2 garlic cloves minced

1 tsp salt
1/4 tsp blackpepper
1 tbsp fresh rosemary chopped
Beet microgreens to serve
4-5 tbsp sunflower hemp crumb to serve (page 23)

Cut the tops and ends of your beets, peel them, wash and cut in two. Place in a pot, cover with water, add 1 tbsp lemon juice or vinegar. This will help to keep the beets from bleeding. Bring to a boil, reduce heat and simmer until tender, about 40- 45 minutes. Once cooked, remove beets from the pot. Keep the beet water to use later for sauteing the onions. The water will keep in a glass jar in the refrigerator up to 4-5 days.
In a non-stick pan, add the chopped onions and garlic. Add 1/4 cup beet water. Saute until soften and caramelized with the beet water (broth). Add more beet water if needed.
Place beets in the pan, toss with the onions, cook on medium for for about 2-3 minutes stirring constantly.
Transfer mixture in a high speed blender. Add the almond milk and salt. Blend until you get a smooth shiny mixture.
Pour mixture in a pot. Cook on medium heat until thicken.
Cook your gluten-free pasta according to the package instructions. Strain and set aside.
Once the beet sauce is thickened, add the pasta, toss well together with the sauce.
Serve with sunflower hemp crumb and beet microgreens.

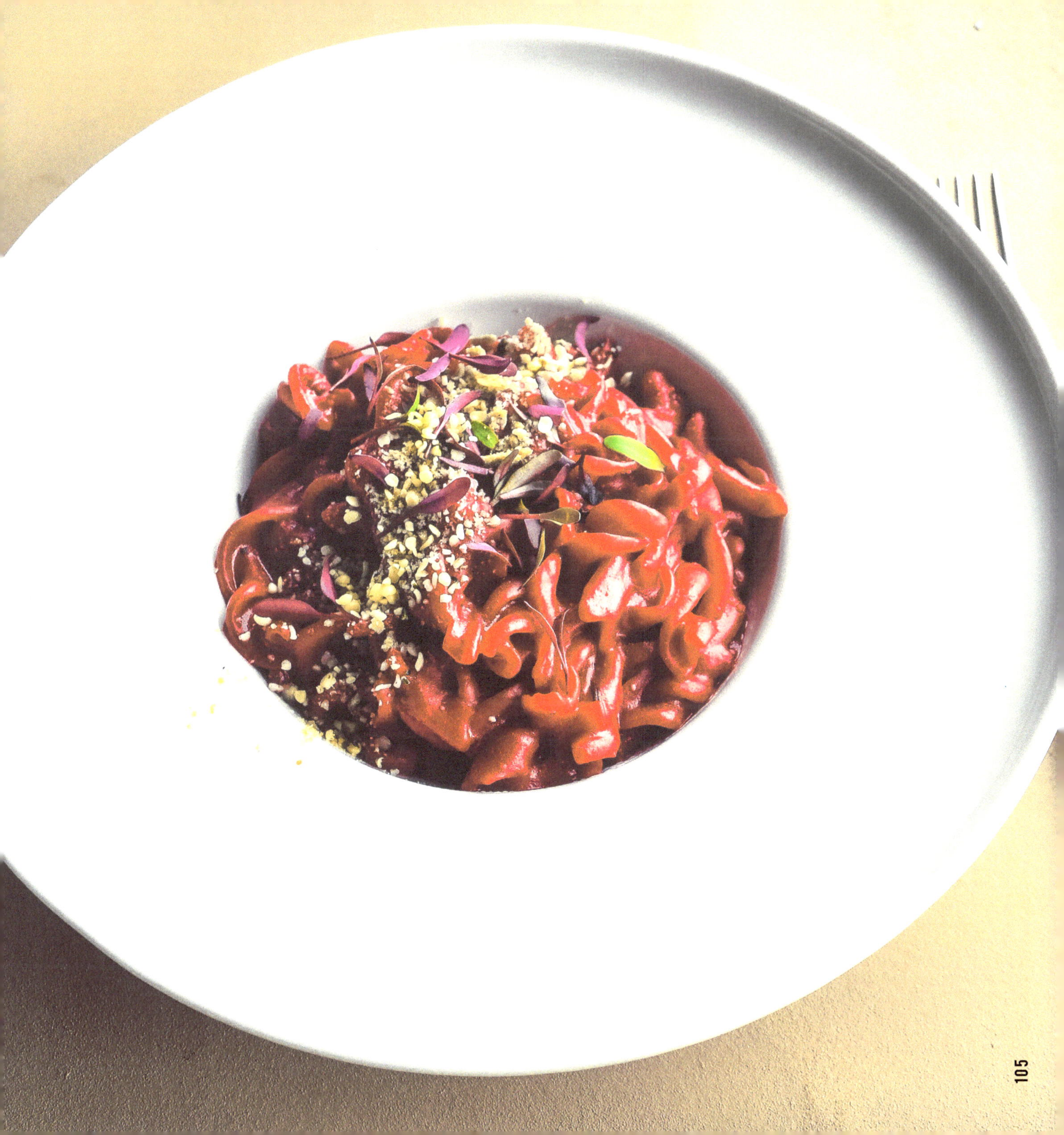

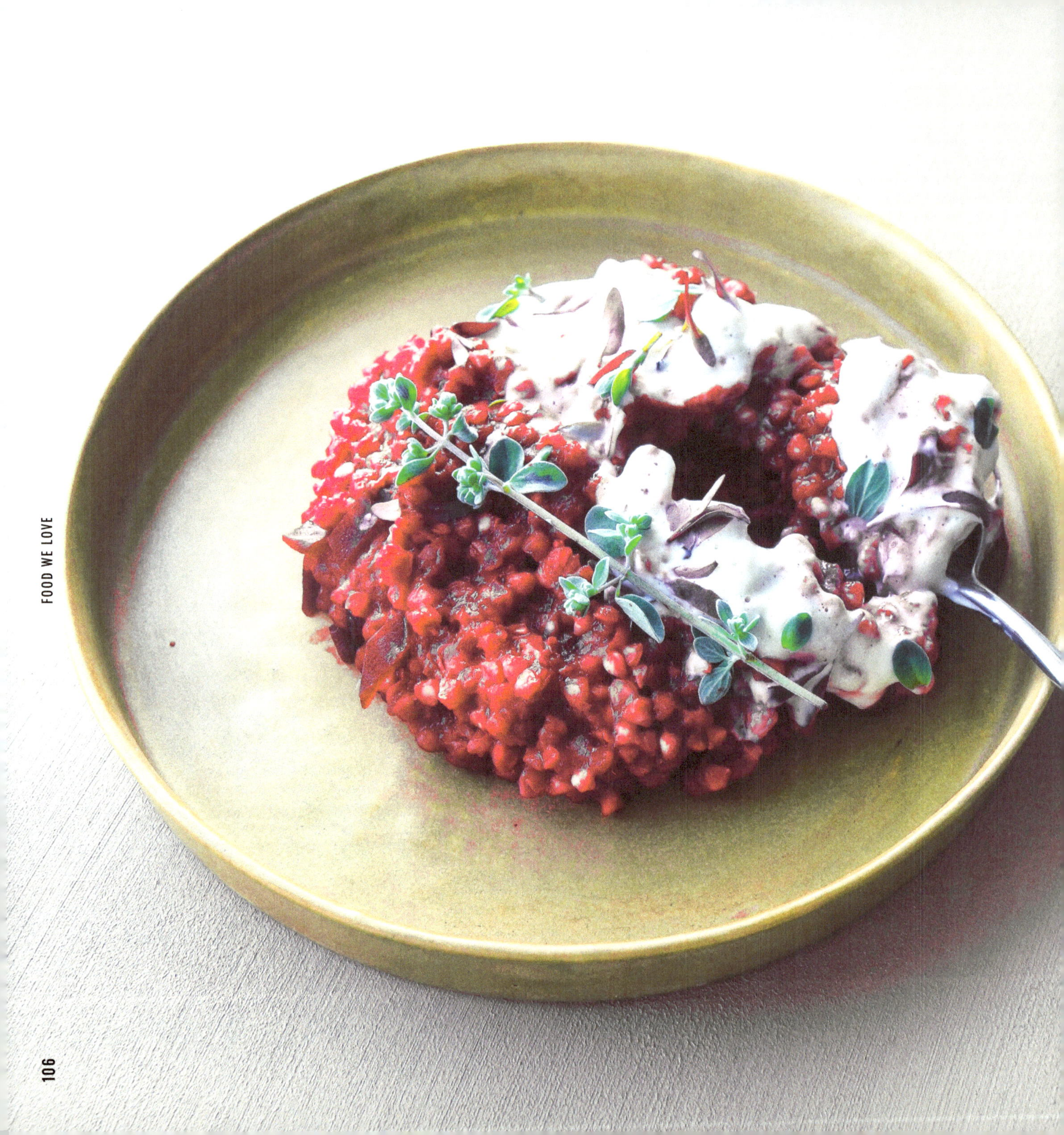

BUCKWHEAT RISOTTO WITH BEETROOT AND YOGURT

Time - 1 hour
Serves - 2-3 person

140 g unroasted buckwheat groats
230 g cooked beetroot
1 medium red onion chopped finely
2 garlic cloves minced
120 ml plant milk
1 tbsp fresh lemon juice
Salt and pepper to taste

Tangy Almond Dressing
90 g blanched almonds soaked (or silken tofu from hemp, soy or oats of your choice)
2 garlic cloves minced
1 tsp dijon mustard
3 tbsp lemon juice
2 tbsp water + more as needed
1/2 tsp salt

Toppings
3-4 tbsp pickled beetroot to serve
Fresh rosemary or majoram
Beetroot microgreens to serve

In a deep pot, put the beetroots, cover with water. Bring to boil until soften enough.
Thoroughly rinse the buckwheat. Drain and set aside.
Once your beets are soften, strain and pour the beet water in a glass bottle to use sautéing the onions.
In a pot, add 3-4 tbsp beet water, add the chopped onions and minced garlic. Sauté on medium heat until onions are soften and caramelized nicely. Then cut your cooked beetroots in small pieces, add to the pot. Toss with the onions and garlic. Cook for 1-2 minutes. Then remove from the heat. Transfer in a high speed blender. Add the plant milk and lemon juice. Process until you get a smooth beetroot puree.
Add the buckwheat in a wide pot, add the beetroot puree, and then cook on a low to medium heat until all the liquid is absorbed (it takes around 15-20 minutes). Keep stirring every 5-6 minutes.
Whilst the risotto is cooking, slice pickled beetroot thinly, then cut into small cubes.
Wash your herbs and microgreens.
Place all the almond dressing ingredients in a blender. Blend until smooth. Pour in a glass and refrigerate at least 1-2 hour before serving.
Once risotto is cooked season with salt and pepper. Sprinkle some pickled beetroot, microgreens and herbs. Top with almond dressing and serve! (Pomegranates also go well with this dish, add some if you like.)

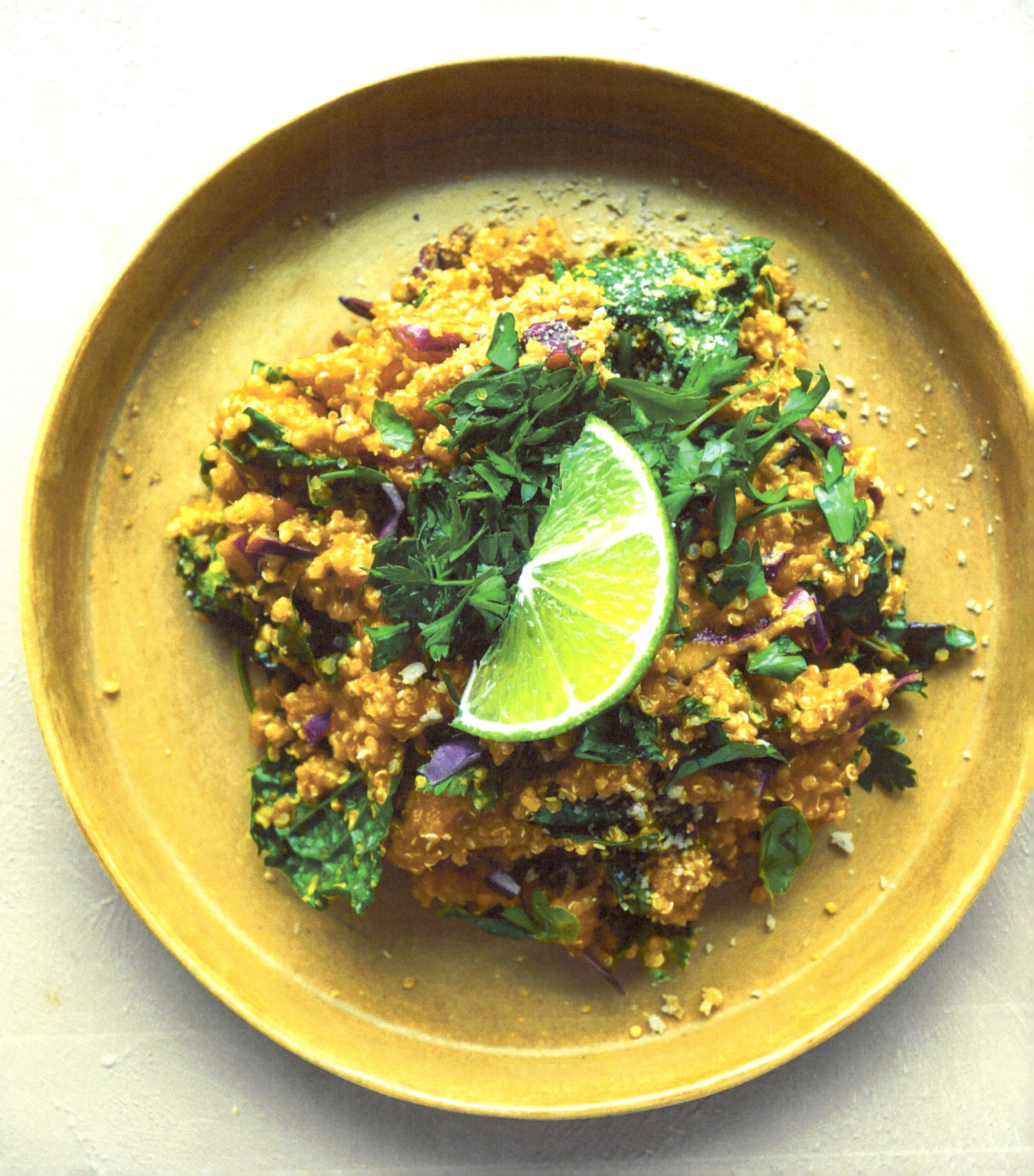

QUINOA WITH CARROT CREAM, KALE, CABBAGE AND PARSLEY GREMOLATA

Time - 40 minutes
Serves - 2-3 person

150 g quinoa
240 ml filtered water
1/2 tsp sea salt
1/4 tsp ground black pepper
100 g dinosaur kale
100 g finely chopped red cabbage
Lime wedges to serve

Carrot cream
400 g carrots (or pumpkin)
1 red bell pepper
1 medium red onion
3 garlic cloves
1/2 tsp sea salt
2-4 tbsp water as needed for creamy consistency
1 tsp red pepper flakes

Parsley Gremolata
1/2 bunch parsley
Juice of whole lemon
2 garlic cloves
A pinch of salt

Pour the water, place a stainless steel steamer basket in the instant pot.
Add the carrots in the basket. Pressure cook at high pressure for 2-3 minutes, then quick release.
Chop your red bell pepper, onion and garlic. In a pot add 2 tbsp water, place the onion and garlic. Cook at medium heat for 3-4 minutes or until onions are soften enough.
Place soften onions and garlic into a high speed blender along with the cooked carrots. Add salt, red pepper flakes and 2 tbsp water. Then blend on high speed until you get a nice smooth carrot cream.
Place your quinoa in a small pot, wash and strain. Cover 1 cup filtered water and cook at medium heat for about 15 minutes or until the quinoa absorbs all the water. Once cooked season with salt and black pepper, set aside.
Wash and cut your kale leaves into small pieces. Preheat a non-stick skillet over medium heat. Once the pan is ready add the kale and cook for a few seconds then add the water to sautee. Cook until the kale starts to wilt and turns bright green.
To make parsley gremolata, remove the stems from the parsley. Chop the parsley with a chef's knife until it is nearly finely chopped. Grate the garlic clove over the parsley. Add fresh lemon juice over the parsley. Toss together.
In a bowl, mix all the ingredients together, coat your quinoa with the carrot cream well. Add the parsley gremolata and cabbage. Serve with lime wedges.

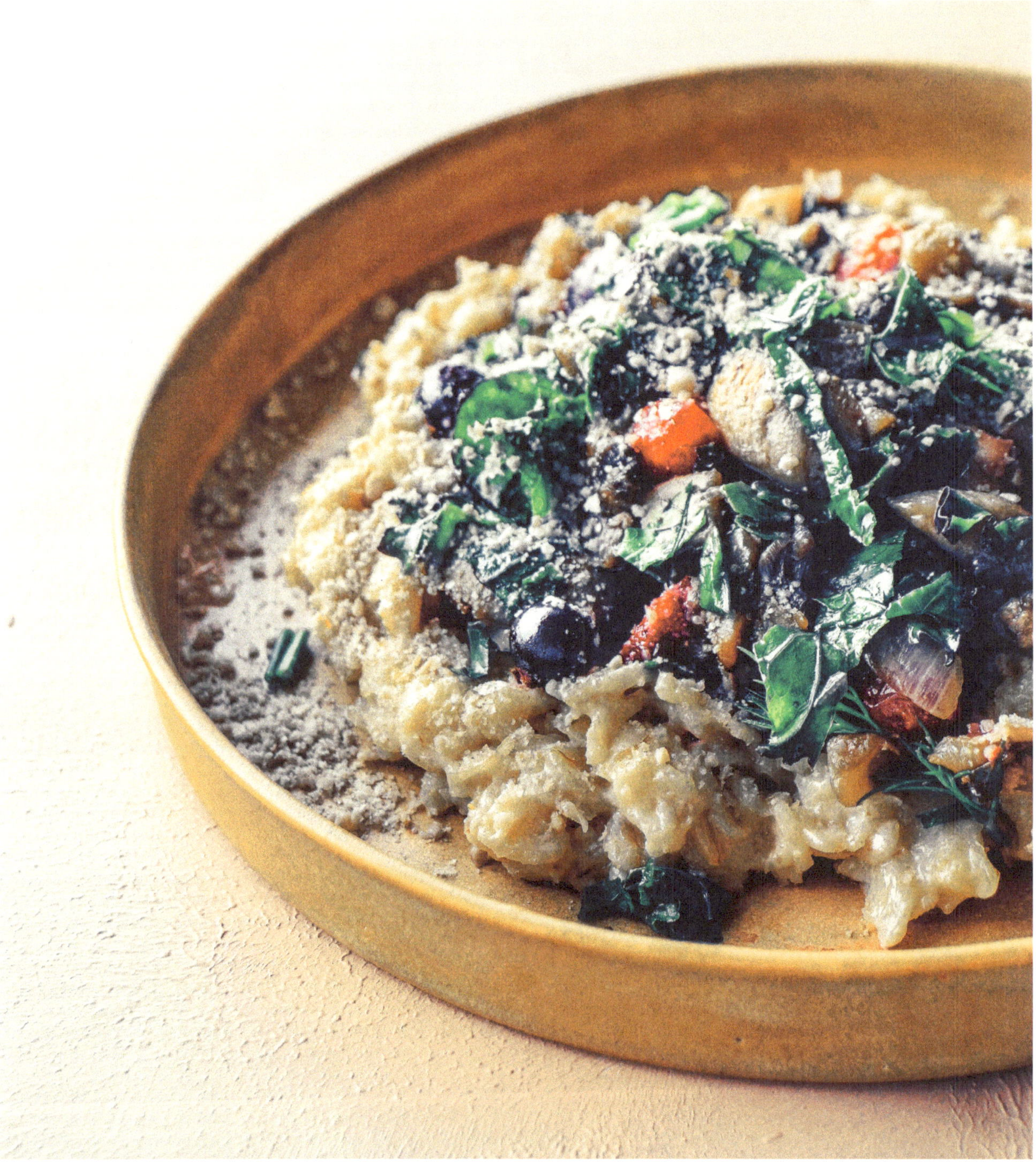

SAVORY OAT PORRIDGE WITH MUSHROOMS, KALE AND BERRIES

Time - 20 minutes
Serves - 2 person

130 g gluten -free rolled oats
600 ml plant milk
2 tbsp beetroot broth or water
1 tsp salt
1 tbsp dried or fresh rosemary (optional)
1 red onion chopped
2 garlic cloves minced
200 g mushrooms (button, cremini, shiitake)
50 g fresh lingonberries, blueberries or your favorite forest fruits
1/2 bunch kale
Nut parmesan to serve

Pour boiling water into the cup of dried rosemary until they are fully covered. Make sure to cover your rosemary with a visible level of water above them. This will ensure that rosemary absorbs the water well and it becomes very soft. Place a lid on top of the glass bowl to maintain the temperature. You can use fresh rosemary as well. If you will not use the herb, skip this step.

Place rolled oats in a pot. Pour the plant milk over the oats. Add the soften rosemary if you are using. Cook until oats absorb the milk and become creamy.

In a pan, put the chopped onions, garlic and mushrooms. Add 2 tbsp beetroot broth or water. Cook on medium heat until caramelized.
Then add the caramelized onions and mushrooms over the cooked oats. Stir well.
Wash and cut your kale leaves into small pieces. Preheat a non-stick skillet over medium heat. Once the pan is ready add the kale and cook for a few seconds then add the water to sautee. Cook until the kale starts to wilt and turns bright green. Top on the oats. Add the berries. Toss together.
Season with salt. Sprinkle some nut parmesan. Taste and adjust the flavour.
Divide between two plates. Serve immediately!

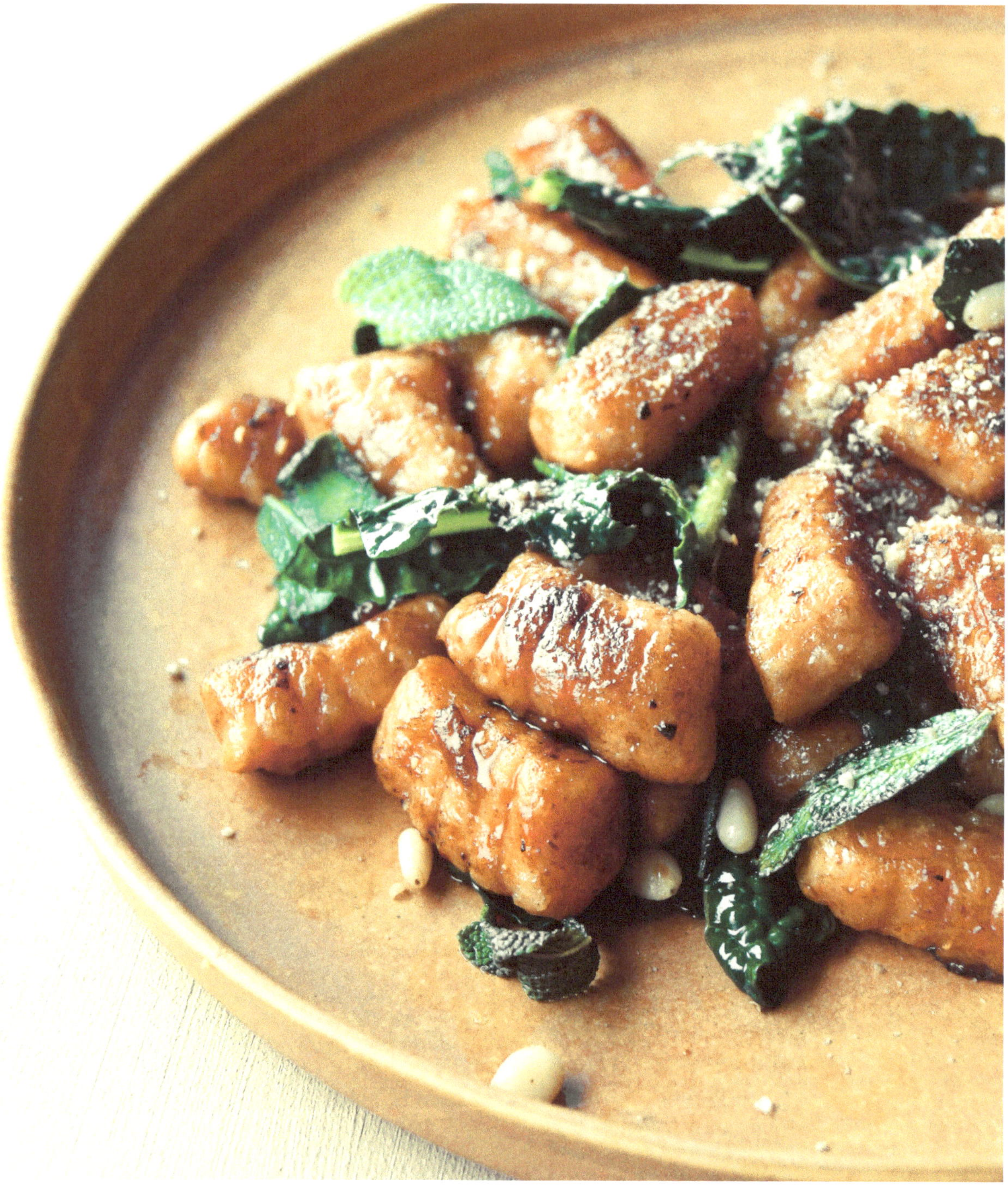

SWEET POTATO GNOCCHI WITH KALE AND SAGE

This sweet potato gnocchi recipe is an autumn-inspired take on gnocchi. Fluffy, tender, and melt in your mouth with a delicious sage and balsamic sauce.

Time - 40 minutes
Serves - 4 person

260 g sweet potato
120 g buckwheat flour
35 g cassava or tapioca flour
60ml water
1 tbsp psyllium husk powder
Salt and pepper to taste

To Serve

150 g kale to serve
2 tbsp lemon juice
2 tbsp balsamic vinegar
Fresh sage leaves to serve
Toasted pine nuts

TIPS

Don't use warm sweet potato! The cooked sweet potato has to be cooled down completely before adding the flours. Why? Because if it is still warm, it will likely absorb more flour and your sweet potato gnocchi will be rather hard and stiff.

Peel and cut the sweet potato, cook in boiling water until soften. The smaller you cut it, the shorter the boiling time is. I found that for 1-inch cubes it takes approx. 10-15 minutes.

Smash the sweet potato with a fork and use your hand to combine it with buckwheat flour, cassava or tapioca, psyllium, water, salt, and pepper. Don't overwork it.

Take a small piece and form long tubes. Keep a good amount of flour close by when you're rolling and cutting your gnocchi – depending on the moisture level of your potato, you may need a sprinkling of it from time to time. Then cut the tubes into inch-long pieces. You can add stripes to your gnocchi by pushing them against a fork. However, if you prefer the authentic traditional gnocchi look, you should get gnocchi strippers.

Cook your sweet potato gnocchi in boiling water. It takes about 1 minute for the gnocchi pieces to rise to the surface. Wait another 2 minutes and you can take them out with a strainer. They will get plenty of time to cook in the pan, so just a couple minutes in boiling water is enough. If you let them get too soft they risk falling apart.

Heat the balsamic in a large frying pan over a medium heat. then add the gnocchi. Cook for 3 mins until starting to brown, then stir in the kale.

Divide gnocchi among 3-4 servings. Pile your gnocchi on top of a bed of lemony kale. Garnish with lemon zest, chopped fresh sage leaves, nut cheese or pine nuts, and any balsamic that may be left in the pan.

WARM GREEN LENTIL SALAD WITH TOMATOES AND AVOCADO

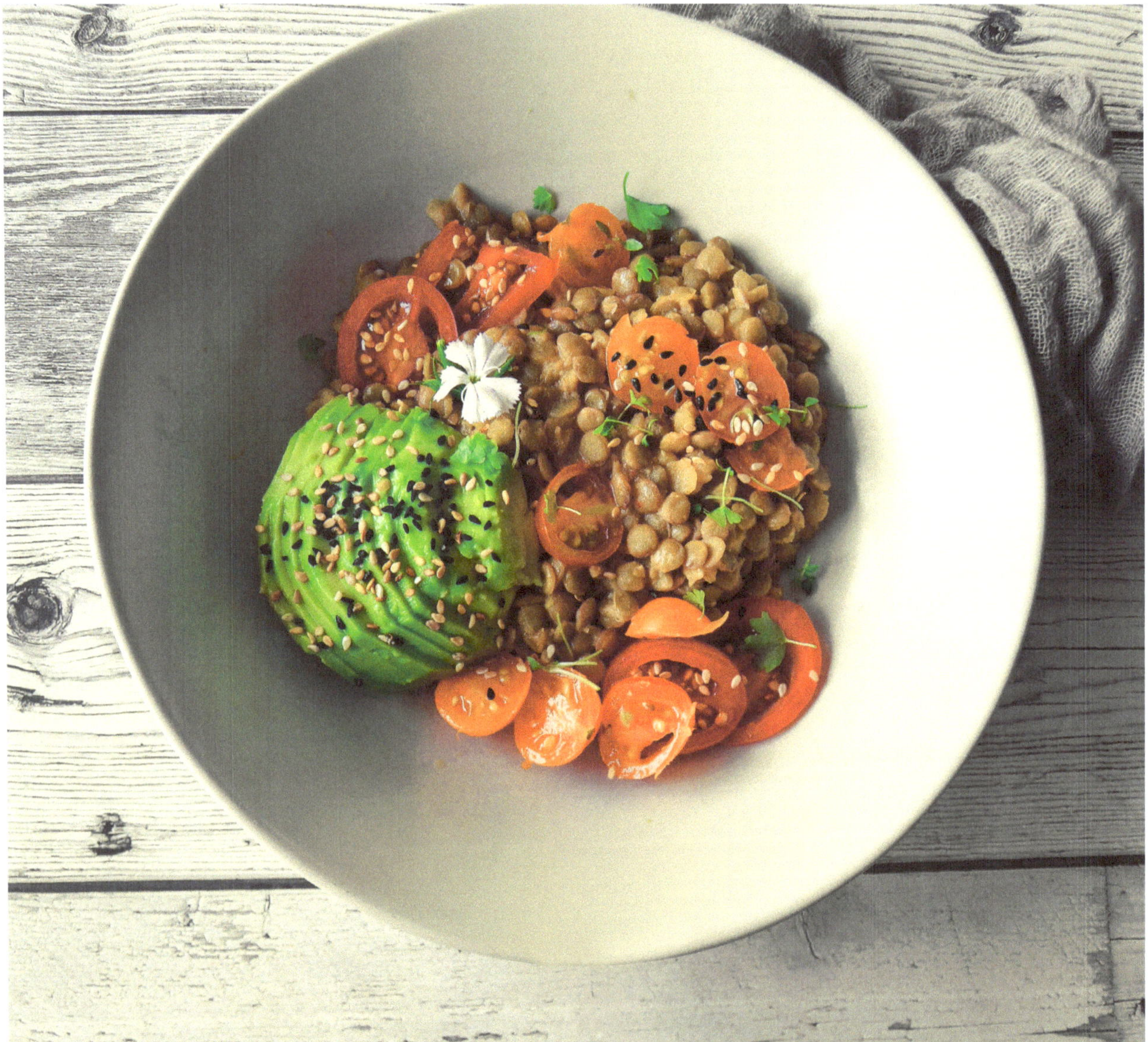

Time - 30 minutes
Serves - 4 person

250 g green lentils
1 yellow onion finely chopped
1 carrot finely chopped
1 celery stalk finely chopped
4 tbsp beetroot broth
A handful of flat-leaf parsley, chopped
1 bay leaf
600 to 700 water as needed
1/2 tsp salt

To serve
2 ripe avocados
2 cups cherry tomatoes
2 small red onion chopped
2 lemon juice
3 garlic cloves minced
Salt as needed

Rinse the lentils well and set them in a bowl. Cover with hot water and soak for at least 15-20 minutes.
Place the onion, carrot, and celery in a large saucepan with 4 tablespoons beetroot broth. Sauté gently on low heat until the vegetables are very soft. Add the bay leaf and the drained lentils and water.
Bring to a boil and then turn the heat down to a gentle simmer and cook until the lentils are tender but retain their shape for about 15-20 minutes. Remove the bay leaf.
Keep checking them and add more water if necessary. Add salt to taste only once the lentils are tender, otherwise they will remain tough.

Stir through chopped parsley and serve with chopped avocados drizzled with lemon garlic dressing, chopped cherry tomatoes, onions or serve as you like. This is very versatile stew.

TIPS
Swap only for beluga. Because green lentils are typically used to make this stew, as beluga and green lentils are firm and retain their shape when cooking. Red or yellow lentils are softer and faster-cooking, with the tendency to fall apart into a thick and wonderful mush when cooked; these are better suited for soup, sauces, or dips.

BUCKWHEAT PASTA WITH BALSAMIC TOMATO SAUCE

Time - 50 minutes

Serves - 4 person

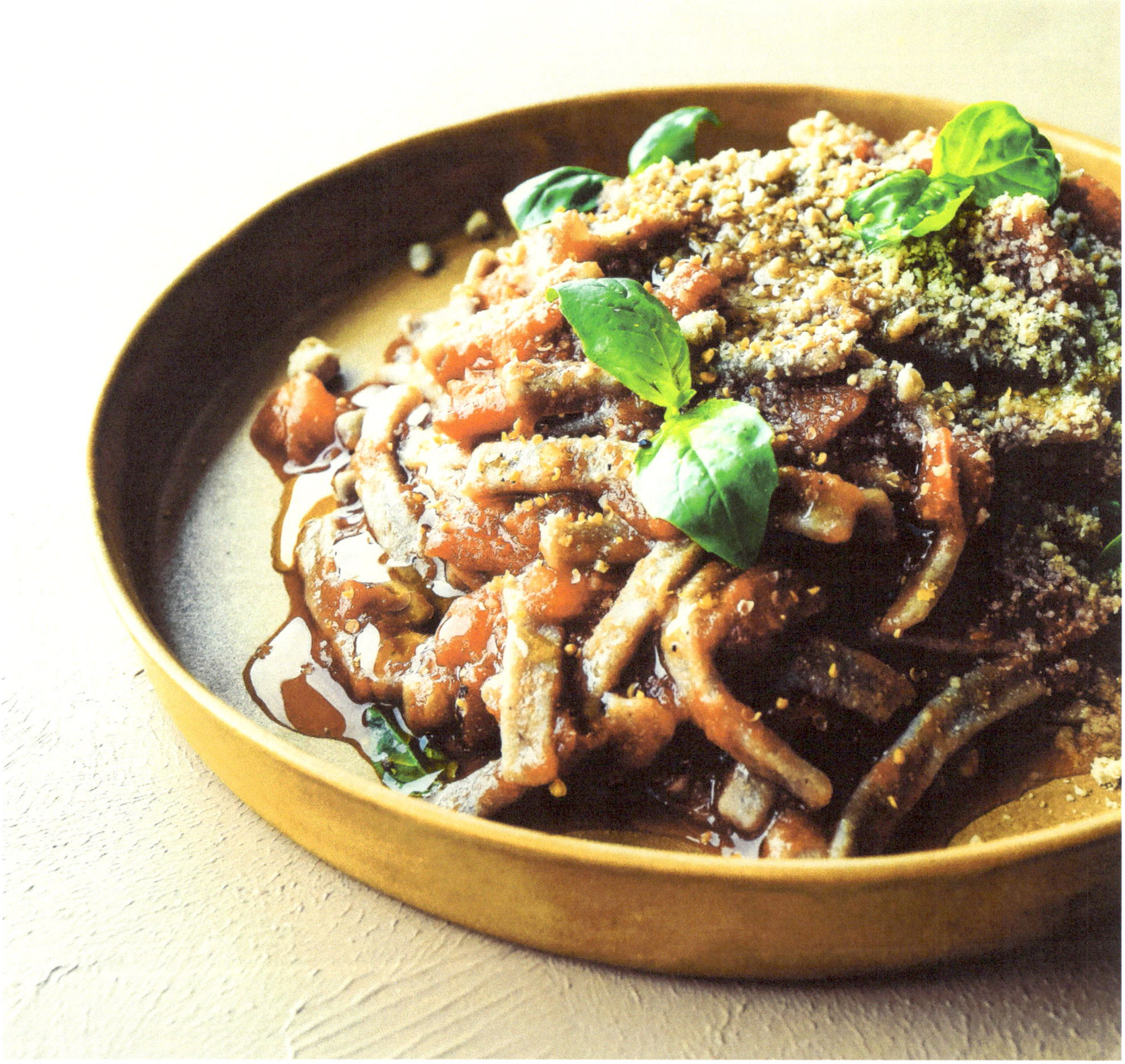

1 cup (120 g) buckwheat flour
1/2 cup (65 g) cassava or tapioca flour
90 ml water
1 tbsp psyllium husk powder + 4 tbsp water
1/4 tsp salt (optional)

In a bowl, whisk together the buckwheat flour, cassava or tapioca, and salt until well-combined.

Add the psyllium, water and start with the first 4 tbsp of water. Mix with a wooden spoon until a nice dough forms. You are looking for slightly moist but not sticky at all.
If your dough is still too dry, add a little more water. At some point you are going to have to ditch the wooden spoon and start using your hands so you can feel the consistency and knead the dough. If it's too sticky add a tablespoon of buckwheat flour until moist but not sticky.
Bring a pot of 8 cups of water and a generous pinch of sea salt to a boil.

Divide the dough into two smooth balls. Flour your surface with more buckwheat flour and roll out one dough ball as thin as you can. You will notice this dough is beautiful to work with! It should be like elastic and easy to roll out.
Using a knife or pizza cutter, create thin strips. Sprinkle with more buckwheat flour to prevent sticking together.

Pour into the boiling water in two batches and cook for approximately 2 minutes. Drain and serve immediately.

Once cooked, this Buckwheat Pasta has a nutty, dense flavor to it but it doesn't stick to your gut the way most pasta does.

It pairs perfectly with simple tomato sauce or balsamic. Simplicity makes this pasta perfection but really, top it with whatever you want. Do be careful with leaving in the strainer for too long. It will start to stick to the other pasta pieces. Make one batch, drain it from the water with a ladle, set it in the strainer and then place into an individual serving bowl immediately. If you find it sticks still, add a small drizzle of balsamic or tomato sauce and lightly separate.

If you will cook the pasta later, dehydrate until completely dried. Keep in the mason jars. You will need to boil dehydrated pasta for 8-10 minutes.
You can dry them at room temperature by hanging in summer days or dehydrate in a food dehydrator at 46° C for 3-4 hours.

Balsamic Tomato Sauce

3 cloves garlic, peeled and sliced
200 g shredded tomatoes
1/2 tbsp tomato paste
1/2 tsp salt
1/2 tsp ground mustard
1 tbsp balsamic
1 tbsp water

In a pot, pour the balsamic and water, add the sliced garlic cloves, cook for 15-20 seconds on medium-high heat until slightly soften. Then add the shredded tomatoes, cook for 1-2 minutes. Then add the tomato paste and continue to cook until thicken. Season with salt and freshly ground mustard. Toss with your pasta and serve immediately.

SQUASH ARTICHOKE SOUP WITH BLACK CAVIAR & BUCKWHEAT CROUTONS

Time - 50 minutes
Serves - 4 person

400 g cretan squash (3 pieces)
6 pieces artichoke hearts, freshly peeled
1 large onion
2 garlic cloves
6 pieces fresh artichoke hearts
Fresh chickweed and purple basil to serve (optional)
Juice of whole lemon
Buckwheat bread for croutons (page 59)

Black Mustard Caviar
1/2 cup black mustard seeds
2/3 cup white wine vinegar
1/3 cup water, plus extra for blanching
2 tbsp grape molasses
A pinch of salt

squash artichoke soup continued

Wash and dry your artichoke and squash.
Cut everything into pieces and steam with garlic and onion.
Place them to a blender, cover with little bit water. As for quantity, you decide: 2 cups or more to make it more or less creamy.
Blend everything using a high speed blender.

Transfer mixture to the pot. Heat on medium heat.
Add the lemon juice, stir well. Serve with black mustard caviar, buckwheat croutons, chickweed and fresh basil leaves.

To make croutons: Cut buckwheat bread (page 59) into small squares, add a pinch of salt in a non-stick pan without adding anything else, toast them until crispy.

To make black mustard caviar, add the mustard seeds to a small pot and cover with enough water. Bring water to a boil, fluffing periodically with a fork to avoid seeds sticking to pan, then remove it from the heat. Drain the water out by pouring the seeds into a mesh strainer and rinsing with cold water. Strain all the liquids out again and repeat this process a couple of times (at least 6 times) to release the bitter tannins from the mustard seeds.
Return the strained seeds back to the pot and add the vinegar, 1/3 cup water, grape molasses and pinch of salt. Bring to a gentle simmer for a few minutes. The seeds should have almost doubled in size and have a somewhat gelatinous texture. Remove from heat and let it cool. Pour into an airtight jar and chill for at least 24 hours before serving.

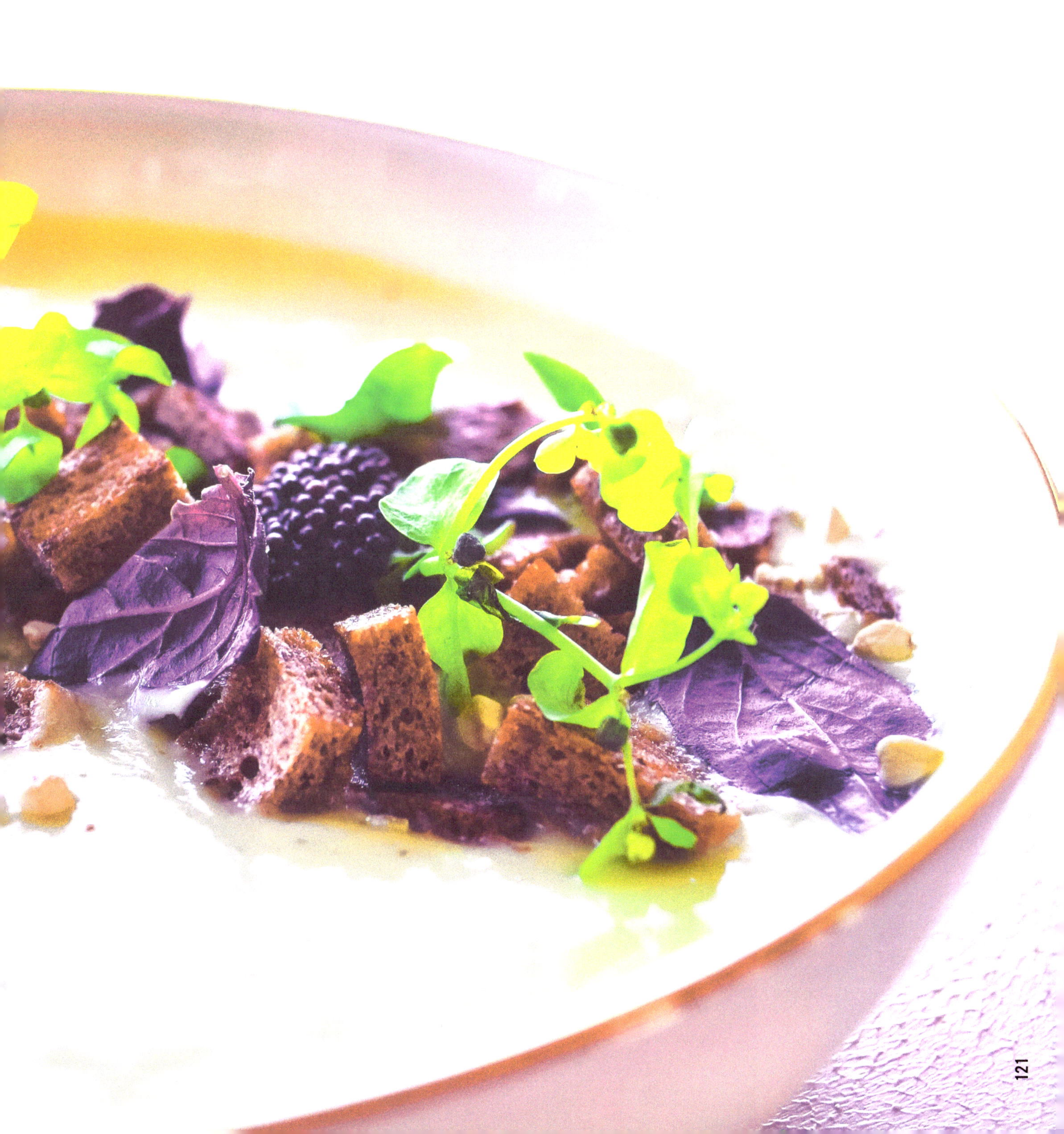

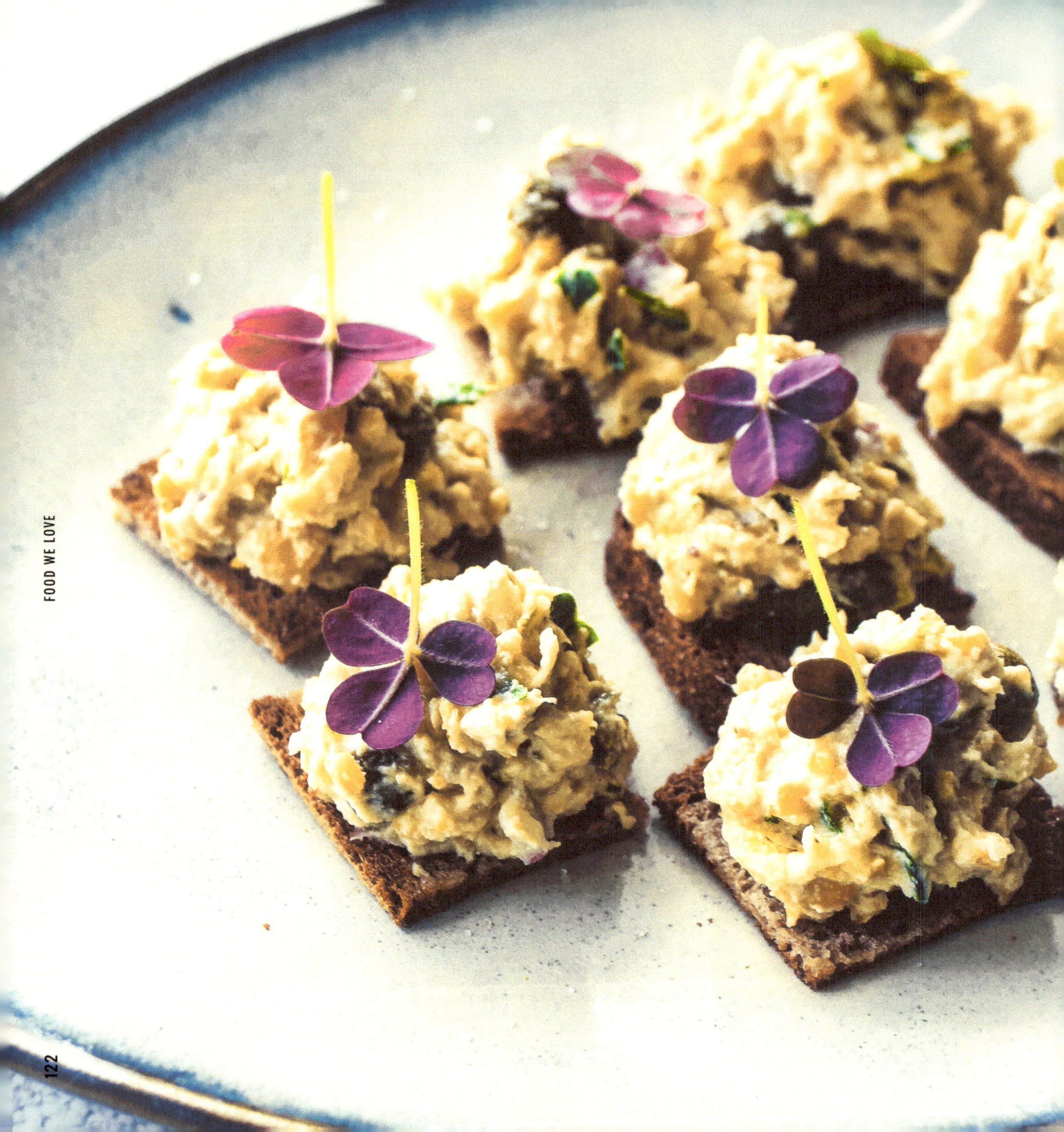

SAVE THE FISH CANAPES

This canapes will give you the mouth feel and fullness that its predecessor, the 'tuna salad' sandwich, gave you. Add some nori sheets or flakes to add more of a sea flavor. This is a wonderful simple mock vegan 'tuna' salad that can be served many ways. Serve on the canapes as I did, spread on your sandwich or scoop on top of a bed of leafy greens with a squeeze of lemon.

Time - 15 minutes
Serves - 4-5 person

400 g cooked chickpeas (canned or cook yourself)
70 g oil-free sunflower seed mayonnaise (just mix the seeds with 3 tbsp lemon juice and water as needed)
1 tsp seaweed blend (nordi,dulse, wakame)
50 g red onion finely chopped
1/2 tbsp djon mustard

2 tbsp capers
50 g chopped celery stalks
1 tbsp lemon juice
1/2 tsp garlic powder
1 tbsp mushroom stock (from dried mushroom water or use tamari, coconut aminos etc)
Salt and black pepper to taste
1/2 tsp apple cider vinegar
1/2 bunch fresh dill
Buckwheat bread for canapes (page 59)

Add the drained and rinsed chickpeas in a large bowl and mash them with a fork.

Add the sunflower seed mayonnaise, finely chopped red onion, seaweed blend, lemon juice, capers, garlic powder, chopped celery stalks, tamari, dijon mustard, dill, white vinegar and salt and pepper. Mix with a fork well.

Taste and add more salt and pepper if needed. Serve chilled or at room temperature. Top on the yeast-free buckwheat bread bites.

Leftovers keep very well in the fridge for 2-3 days.

For the omega addition: Add 1 tablespoon or so of hemp hearts or chia seeds to the no-tuna mix for augmented nutrients.

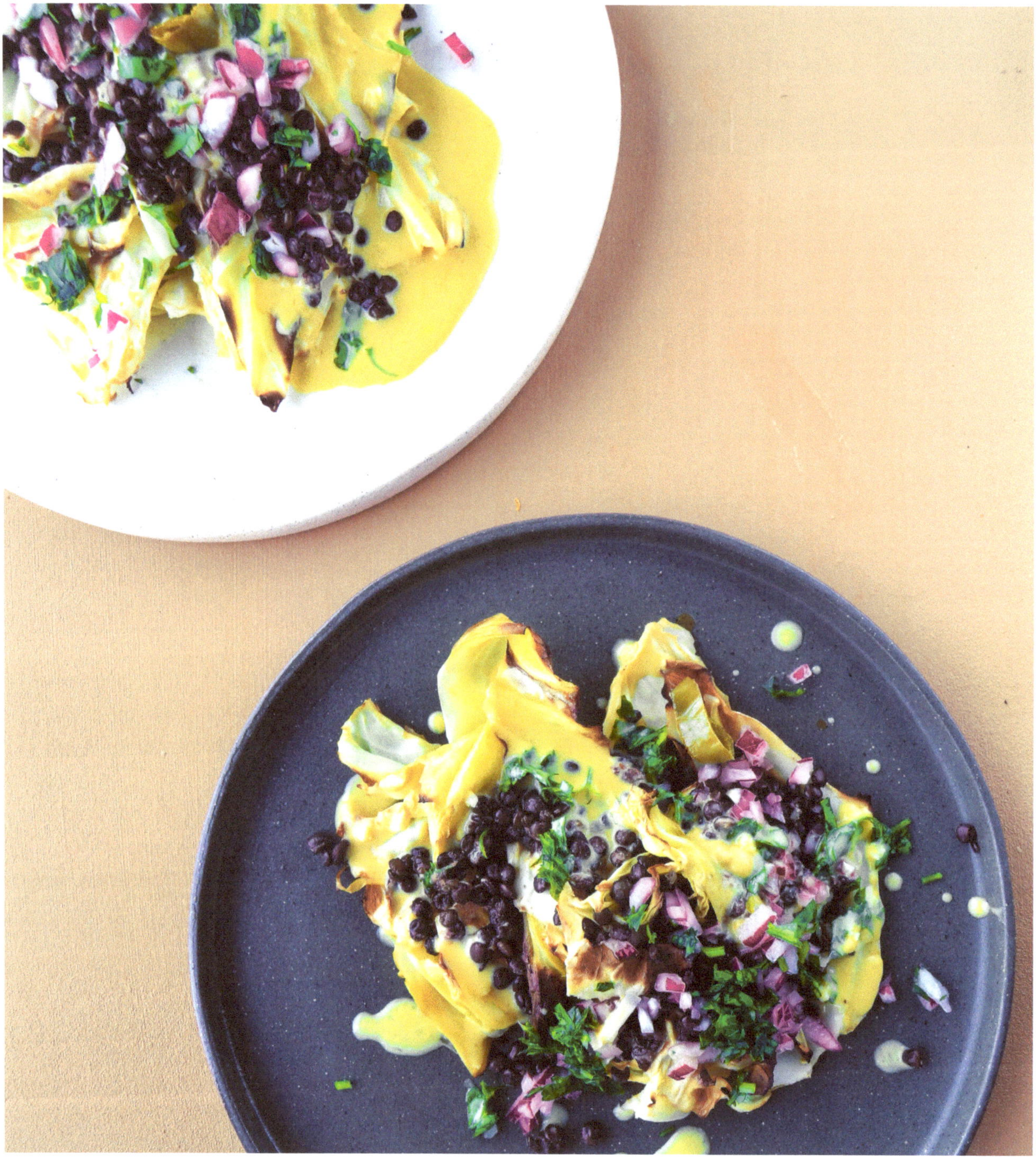

ROASTED CABBAGE WITH MUSTARD SAUCE AND BELUGA

Time - 30 minutes
Serves - 4 person

1/2 medium green cabbage
1/4 cup vegetable broth
Salt and pepper to taste
Lemon wedges to serve
Chopped parsley to serve
Cooked beluga to serve (1 cup beluga cooked in 1 3/4 cup mushroom stock page-30)

Mustard Sauce
Juice of 2 whole lemon
1 medium red onion minced
2 garlic cloves minced
2 tbsp dijon mustard
1/4 tsp salt

Preheat oven to 220° C. Line a baking sheet with parchment paper.
Cut the cabbage half into four equal wedges and set on prepared baking sheet. Use a pastry brush to coat the cut side of each wedge with vegetable broth and sprinkle with salt and pepper. Turn wedges and repeat.

Place the baking sheet in the oven and cook for 10-12 minutes. Flip the wedges and roast until nicely browned, 8-10 minutes more.

Meanwhile, make the sauce by adding all the sauce ingredients to a small bowl and mix until combined well.

Cook the beluga until absorbs all the water.

To serve, place the wedges on a plate, whisk sauce again and drizzle over wedges. Add 2-3 tbsp beluga lentils over the cabbage. Sprinkle some chopped red onion and parsley. Serve with lemon wedges.

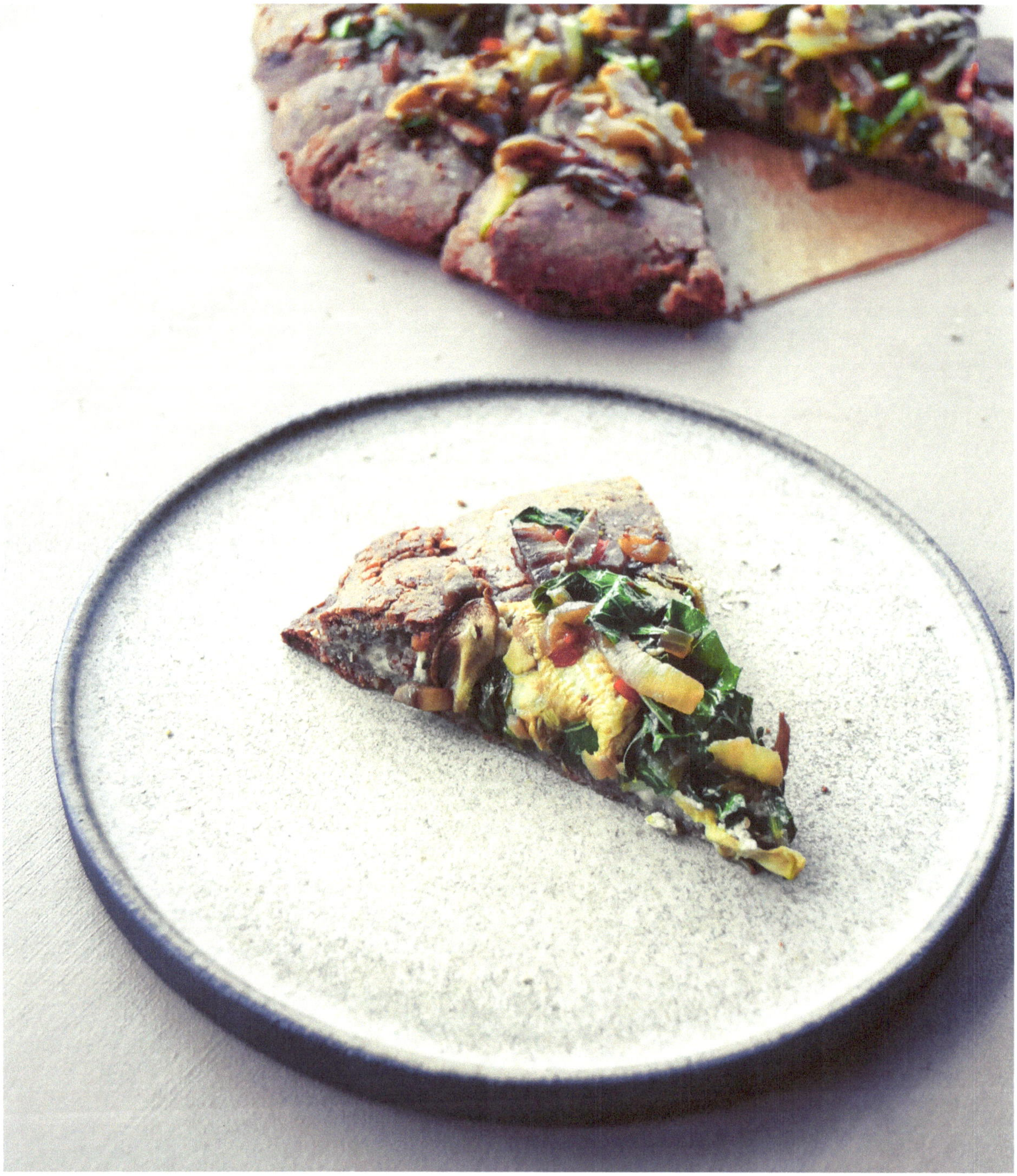

ALMOND GALETTE WITH ZUCCHINI

Time - 40 minutes
Serves - 4 person

For the Galette
130 g almond flour
70 g cassava or tapioca flour
1 tbsp maple
1/4 tsp salt
50 g almond butter
1 tbsp psyllium powder
5 tbsp water
2-3 tbsp plant-based milk to brush the galette

Filling
130 g sunflower seeds
2 tbsp lemon juice
200 ml water
4 garlic cloves minced
1/2 tsp salt
1/4 tsp pepper
1 tsp dijon mustard

Toppings
2 large roasted courgettes
200 g sauted mushrooms
1 cup wilted collard greens (or kale, spinach)

Preheat the oven to 200° C.
To make filling, place all the filling ingredients in a high speed blender, blend until smooth. Set aside.

To make dough, in a mixing bowl, mix the almond flour, cassava, salt and psyllium together. Then add the almond butter, maple and water. (Add 1 teaspoon of water at a time or more, if needed, to make sure the dough comes together) Stir to mix.
Then knead with your hands.
Once the dough is formed, shape it into a ball.
Roll the dough into a circle and add your prepared filling in the middle, leaving a 1-inch border along the sides.
Fold the edges over carefully, brush the pastry with plant milk and then transfer galette into the oven.

Place a large piece of baking paper on the counter, sprinkle it with almond flour. Transfer the galette into the oven and bake for 25 minutes, or until golden brown. Let cool for 10 minutes.

Meanwhile, slice the zucchini lengthwise as thinly as you can.
Brush with vegetable broth before arranging on a griddle pan.
Leave it alone for a few minutes and once the char marks appear on one side, flip it over and char on the other.

Season and set aside. Then top with sauted mushrooms, grilled zucchini, greens or your favorite pesto.
Simply slice it as if it were a pizza and serve as an appetizer or main course. Try pairing it with a salad for an even fuller meal!

CRISPY POTATOES WITH MEXICAN BEANS AND GUACAMOLE

Time - 1 hour

Serves - 3-4 person

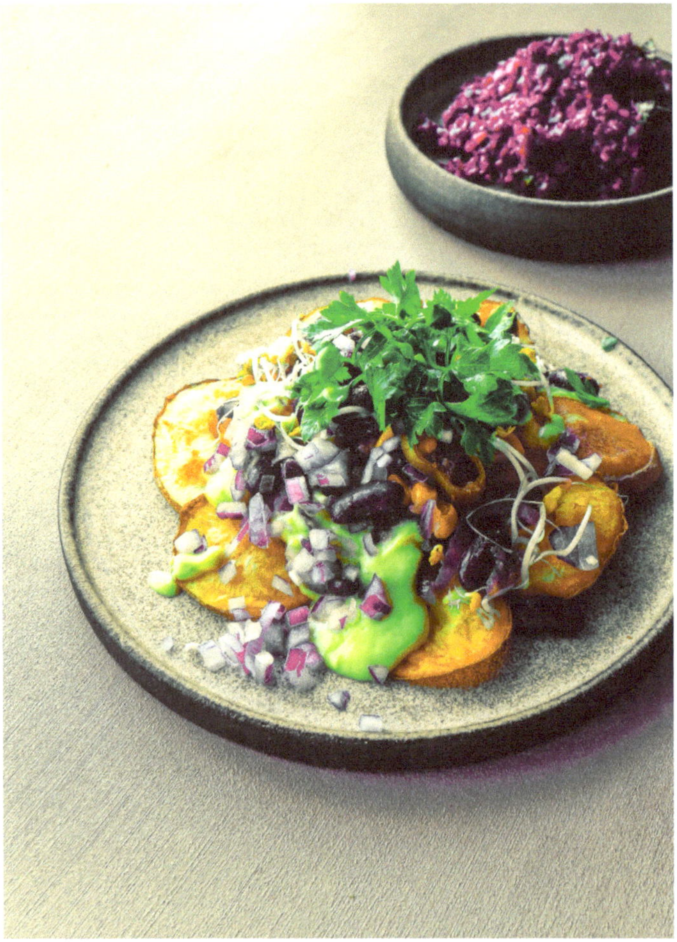

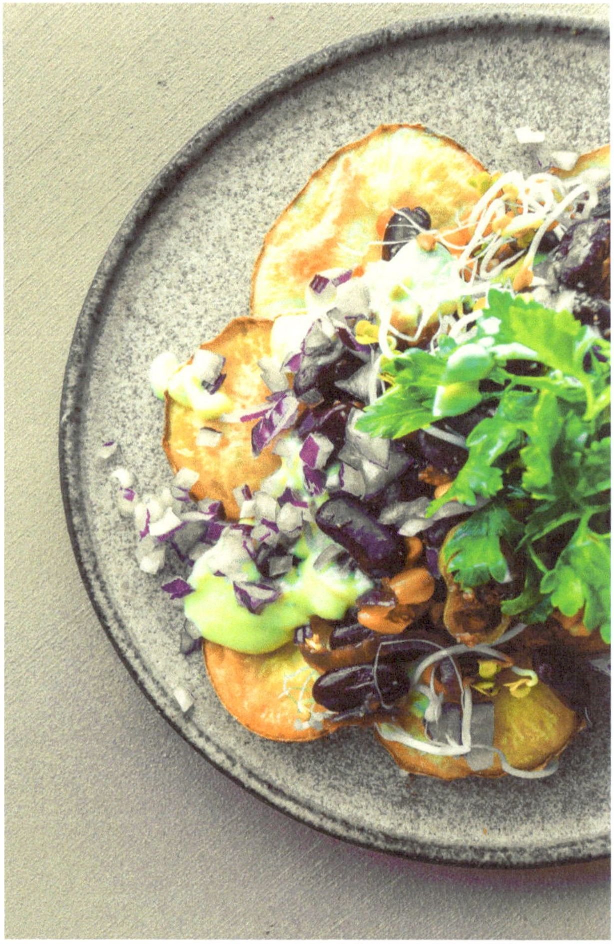

700 g potatoes
180 g mexican beans cooked
3-4 tbsp beetroot broth
1/4 cup cooked corn
1/2 tsp baking soda
1/2 tsp salt
1 tsp chili
2 jalapeños thinly sliced
1 medium red onion finely chopped + more to serve
1/4 bunch fresh parsley chopped
Microgreens to serve

Guacamole

1 ripe avocado
1 garlic clove minced
3 tbsp lemon juice
1/2 tsp salt
1 tbsp water
1/2 jalapeño

Preheat oven to 200º C.

Wash and using a mandoline slicer, slice your potatoes. Place the potatoes in a pot, cover with water. Add 1 tsp baking soda and 1 tsp salt. Bring to boil for about 10 minutes. This process will make your potatoes crispier without oil. Then strain the water. Add some salt as you need. Give it a good toss.

Transfer the potatoes onto a baking tray lined parchment paper.
Bake in the oven for 25-30 minutes or until crispy enough and golden.

To prepare mexican beans, place the cooked beans in a pan, add the corn, beet broth, beans, onion, chili, salt and pepper, cook on medium heat until thick.

To make guacamole, mash your avocado, add the lemon juice, chopped onions, jalapeño, parsley, garlic and salt. Mix well using a fork.

Place your baked potatoes in the plate, add the mexican beans along with the chopped fresh red onion, microgreens, parsley and top with guacamole. Enjoy!

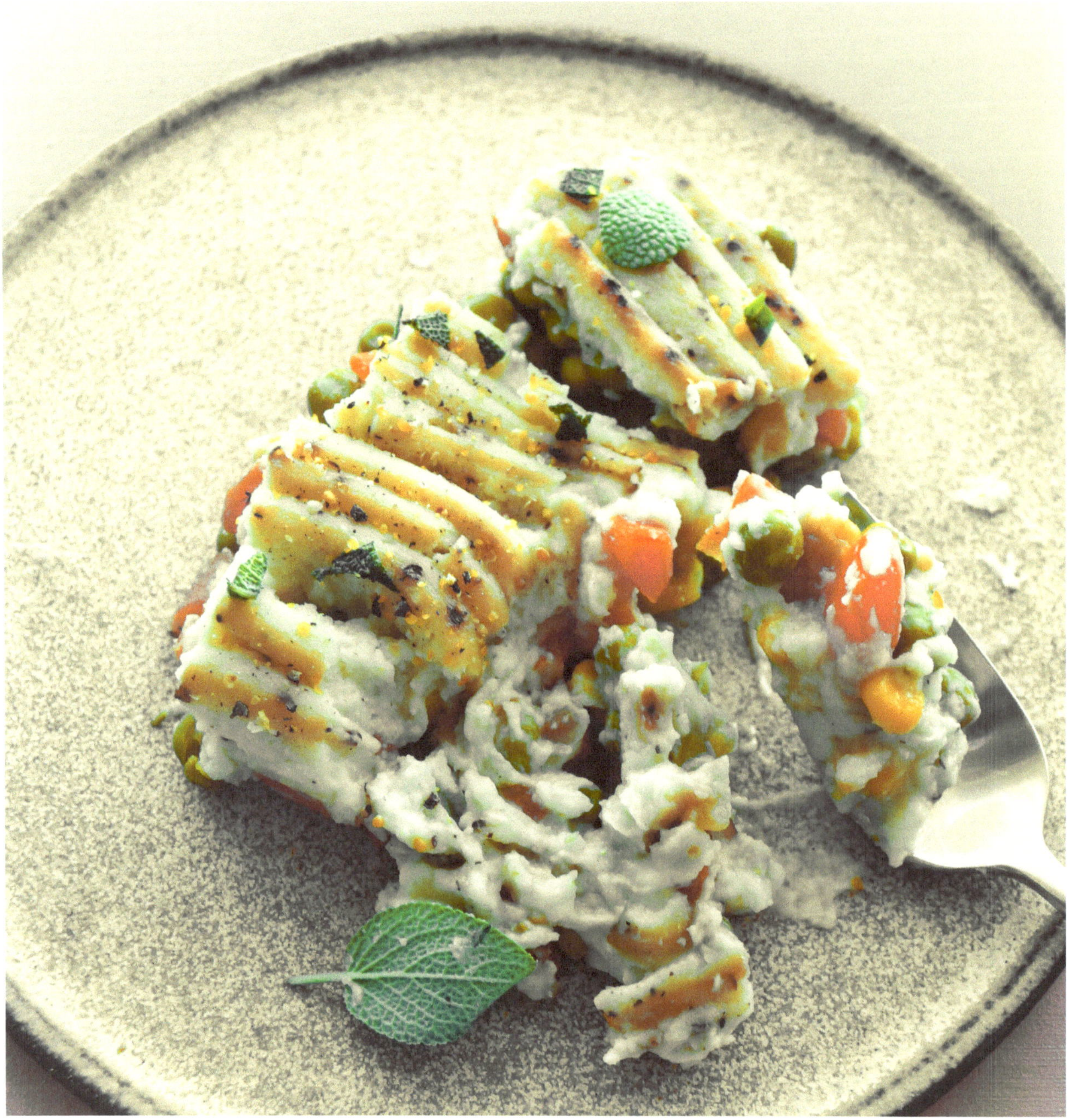

CAULIFLOWER SHEPHERD'S PIE WITH PEAS

Time - 1 hour
Serves - 4-6

1 medium cauliflower cut into florets (approximately 1-1.2 kg)
350 ml almond milk (blend 350 ml water + 6 blanched almonds together)
1/2 tsp freshly ground black pepper
1 tsp salt as needed
1/4 tsp ground nutmeg
Fresh sage leaves chopped to top

Filling
2 medium yellow onions chopped
3 garlic cloves minced
2 cups fresh or frozen green peas
1/4 cup heirloom corn
4 medium carrot diced
1/4 cup beetroot broth
1/4 cup mushroom broth
1/2 tsp ground bay leaf
1/2 tsp salt

Place the cauliflower florets into a medium sized saucepan and cover with 1 quart of water. Bring water to a boil over high heat. Reduce heat. Boil at a simmer for 5-7 minutes until the cauliflower is fork tender.

Once done, strain the excess water, transfer the cauliflower to a high speed blender.
Add the almond milk, black pepper, nutmeg and salt. Blend until smooth puree. Set aside.

In a large pan, add the garlic, onions and beetroot water. Saute until absorbs the water and soften. Then add the carrots, peas, corn and bay leaf. Pour the mushroom broth over the veggies. Cook until absorbs the water.

Preheat oven to 220° C.
Once the veggie mixture is cooked, taste and adjust seasonings as needed. Then transfer to your prepared oven-safe baking dish and carefully top with cauliflower puree. Smooth down with a spoon or fork and season with another crack of pepper and a little sea salt.
Place on a baking sheet to catch overflow and bake for 35-40 minutes or until the mashers are lightly browned on top.
Let cool briefly before serving. The longer it sits, the more it will thicken. Let cool completely before covering, and then store in the fridge for up to a few days.

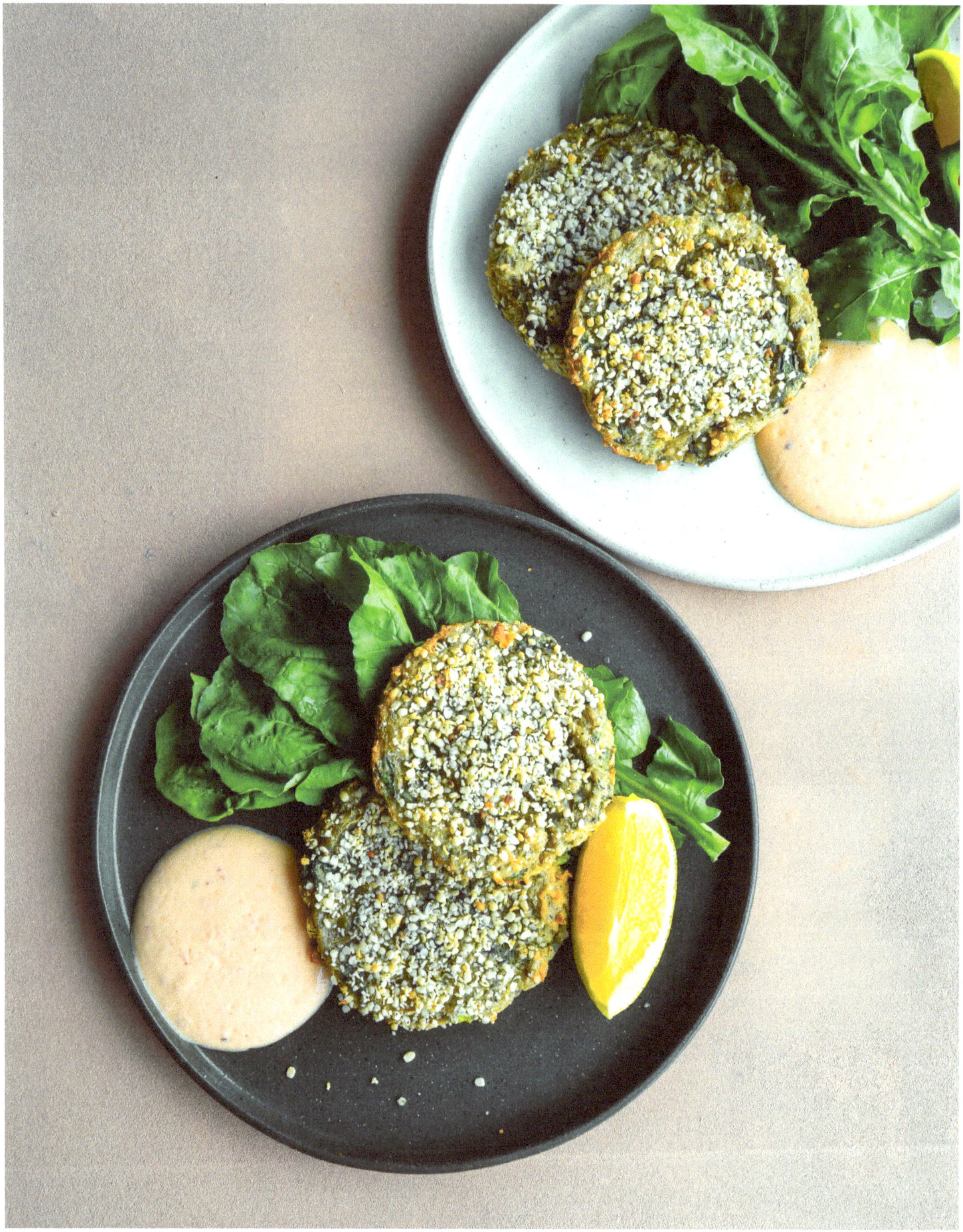

CRAB CAKES WITH RED BELL PEPPER AILOI

These nutty crab cakes are full of umami flavours that merge sour, salty, and bitter. For a filling meal, serve with rocket greens or salad with lemon wedges.

Time - 50 minutes
Serves - 4 person

400 g potatoes cooked mashed
200 g artichoke meat cooked mashed (or cooked mashed celeriac)
200 g maitake mushrooms chopped
2 spring onions finely chopped
1 tbsp nori powder
1 tbsp capers
1/2 tsp white pepper
1/2 tsp cayenne
Juice of 1/2 lime
100 g buckwheat flour
25 g flaxseeds
Rocket greens and lemon wedges to serve
1/4 cup hemp hearts to coat

Red Bell Pepper Aioli

100 g silken tofu (from soy, hemp or oats) - you can also use cashews or almonds if you prefer.
35 g red bell pepper
3 garlic cloves minced
1 tsp dijon mustard
2 tbsp lemon juice
1/2 tsp salt
1/2 tsp chili

Cook and mash the artichoke and potatoes. Set aside.
Chop the maitake mushrooms, spring onions and capers and place in a large mixing bowl. Add in the lime juice, cayenne, nori and white pepper. Stir and add in the chopped parsley. Then add in the mashed potatoes and artichoke.
Grind the flaxseeds and mix well into buckwheat flour. Add in the bladder wrack. Set to one side for about 20 minutes.

Line a tray with parchment paper.
Take a small handful of the mixture make into a round circle to form a cake. Coat with hemp hearts. Place on the parchment paper. Keep repeating till you use up the mixture.
Cook the crab cakes in an air fryer at 185° C for 10 minutes, in batches or in the oven until golden brown. An air fryer gives these cakes a slightly drier yet crunch texture in the centre. If you don't have an air fryer, you can bake in the oven but you will get a softer centre.

To make red bell pepper aioli, place the all red bell pepper aioli ingredients in a high speed blender. Process until smooth. Pour in a glass jar. Refrigerate for about 2 hours before serving.

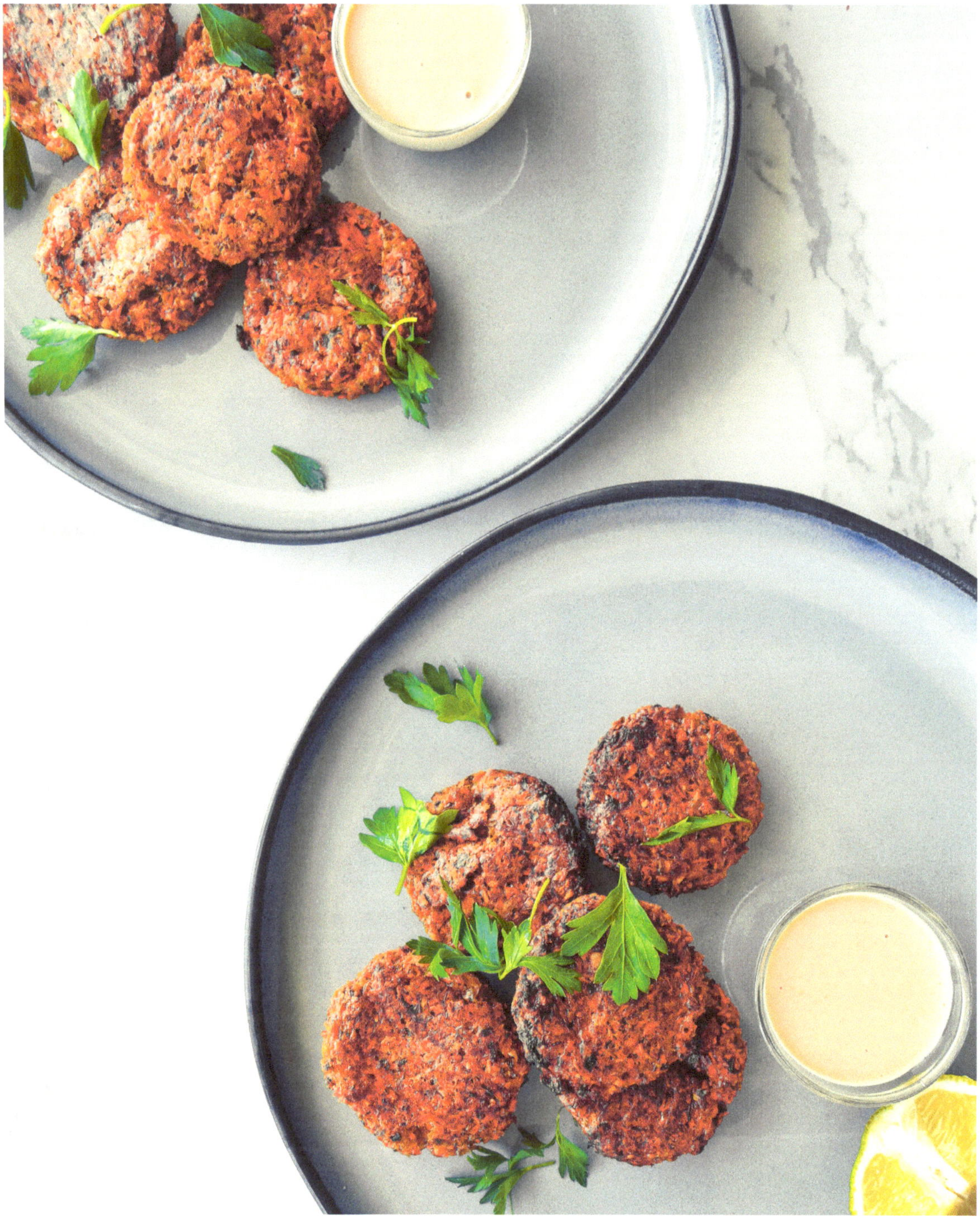

BEET PATTIES WITH TAHINI DRESSING

Time - 30 minutes
Serves - 4 person

360 g beetroot
3 springs green onion
200 g oat or buckwheat flour
A handful of fresh parsley
3 inch freshly grated ginger
2 tbsp balsamic
1 tbsp psyllium husk powder
1 tbsp chia seeds + 3 tbsp water
1/2 tsp salt
Lemon wedges to serve
Fresh parsley chopped to serve

Tahini Dressing
100 g tahini
100 ml water
Juice of 1 whole lemon
1 garlic clove minced
A pinch salt

Preheat oven to 210° C.
Place beets, onions, parsley and ginger in a food processor, mix until well chopped well.
In a small bowl mix chia seeds and water, set aside for 10 minutes until chia absorbs the water and the mixture becomes sticky.
Once done, transfer chia mix into your food processor. Add the oat flour, psyllium husk, balsamic and salt. Continue to mix.
Let it sit in the food processor for 15-20 minutes until they become easy to hold together.

Shape them with your hands into about 15-20 balls.

Bake at 210° C for 35-40 minutes, then flip up and continue to bake until golden brown and crispy enough.

Mix the tahini dressing ingredients in a bowl.
Serve your patties with parsley, lemon slices and tahini dressing. Combine with potatoes or salad for a filling meal.

AMARANTH & BELUGA LENTIL PATTIES WITH CARROTS

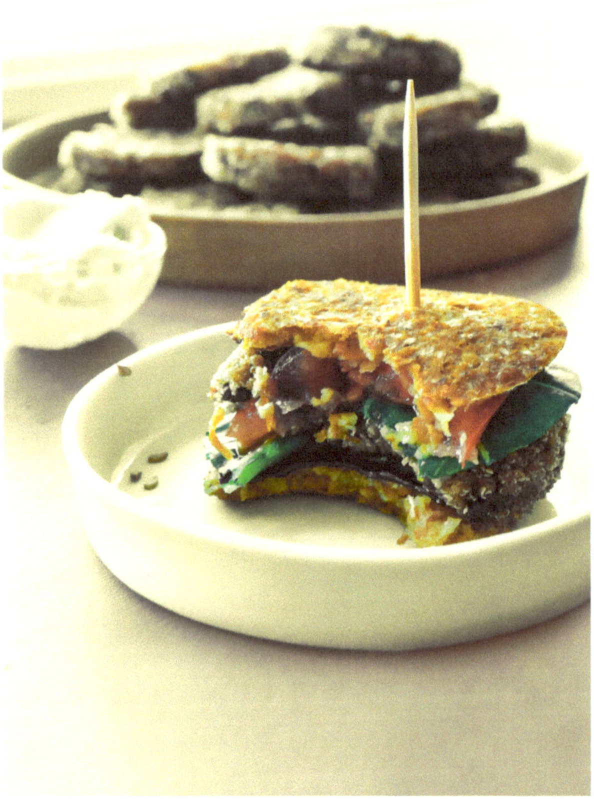

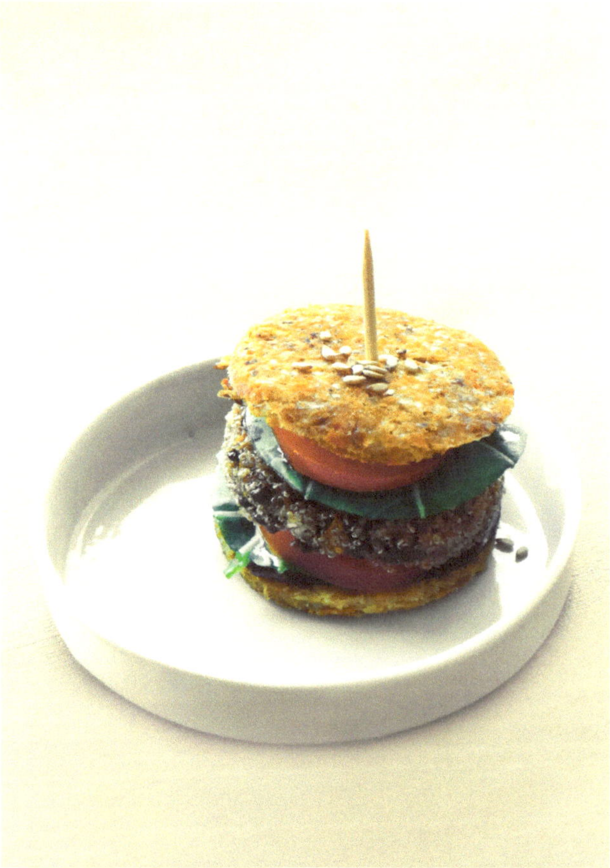

A satisfying patty has to have enough bite to act as the centrepiece of the sandwich or bun, but also has to be juicy. Amaranth grain- a staple food of the Aztecs, takes in lots of moisture as it cooks and holding onto it to create a juicy centre to the burger. It must also have a crispy outside, which can be achieved by baking in the oven without oil. The result is a satisfying, filling patty with a crunchy outer layer, which reveals a firm and juicy centre. It's full of healthy fibre, magnesium and iron which will help to keep you feeling full.

Time - 1 hour 20 min.
Serves - 26 patties

115 g cooked beluga
265 g cooked amaranth
100 g gluten-free bread crumbs (page 156)
1 tbsp psyllium husk powder
75 g carrots thinly shredded
50 g red onion finely chopped
1/4 bunch parsley finely chopped
3-4 tbsp mushroom stock (or coconut aminos or tamari)
4 garlic cloves minced
1 tsp red pepper flakes
1 tsp salt

TIPS

GF Bread crumb substitute can be chickpea flour.

Place cooked beluga, gluten-free bread crumbs, psyllium, carrots, onion, mushroom stock, garlic, parsley, red pepper flakes and salt in a bowl. Stir to combine together.

Then add the cooked amaranth and mix together. Let it sit for 5 minutes. Then using your hands, knead the mixture in the bowl until becomes sticky and everything holds together.

Preheat oven to 200° C.
Line a baking tray with parchment paper.
Using 4-5 cm round cutter with handle, shape the dough. Make small patties, place on the parchment paper leaving 2 cm space between. Repeat the process for the rest.
Bake in the oven for 20-30 minutes, then flip the patties, continue to bake other side for another 20-30 minutes or until golden brown.
Serve with almond cream and your favorite salad for a filling meal or try it packed into sandwich or buns with cauliflower bread (page 57), red onion, tomatoes or iceberg lettuce.

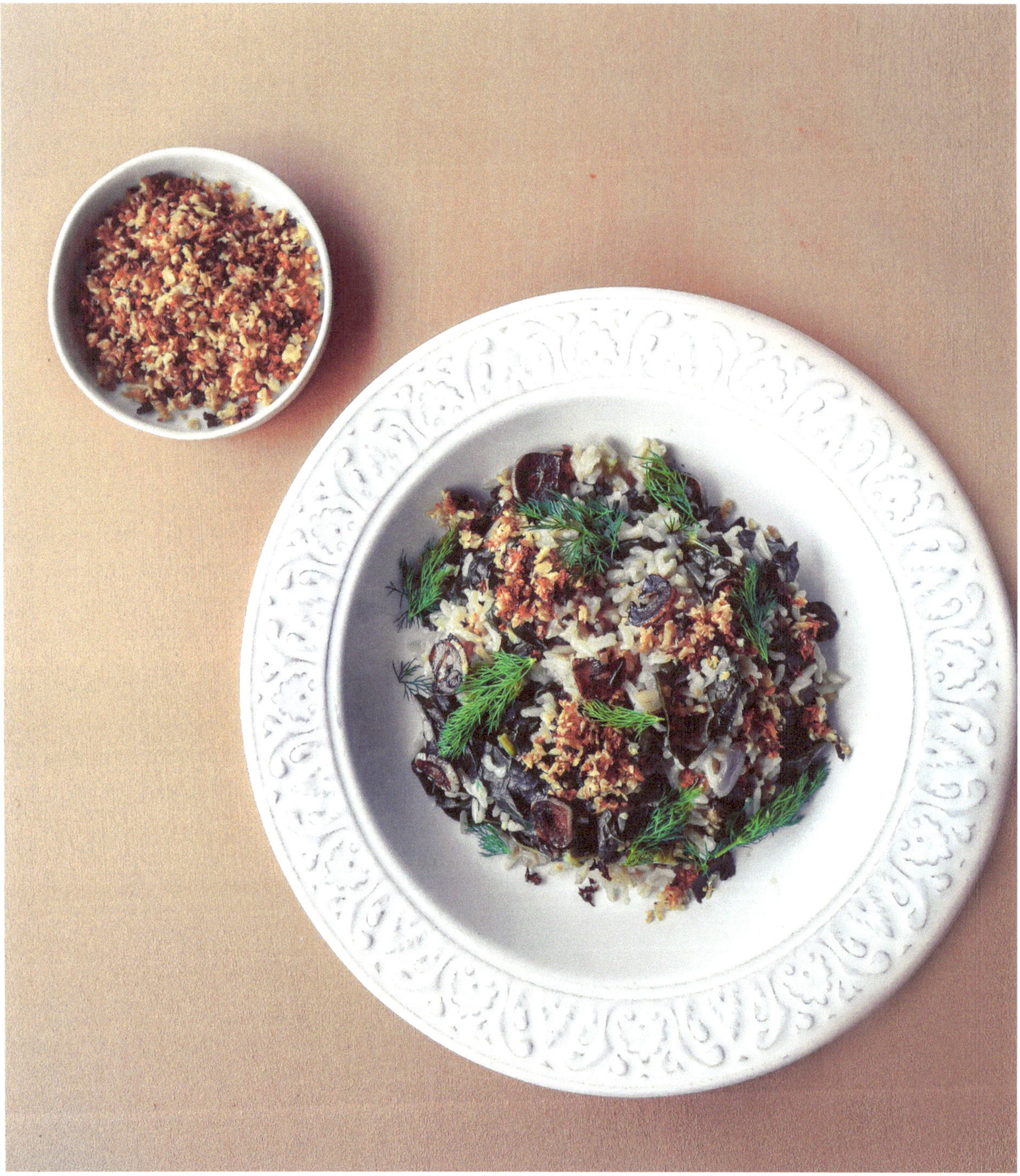

COLLARD WITH BROWN RICE, BALSAMIC GARLIC, CELERIAC CRUMB AND DILL

Time - 40 minutes
Serves - 4 person

500 g collard greens (or kale, spinach, chard etc.)
100 g brown rice +125 ml water
1 onion finely chopped
8-10 garlic cloves thinly sliced + 1 tbsp balsamic + 1 tbsp water
1/4 cup beetroot broth
1 tsp salt
1 tsp chili flakes
1/4 tsp black pepper
1/4 bunch fresh dill
Celeriac crumb to serve (page 23)

Soak your rice overnight. In the morning rinse and dry. Place in a pot. Add the chopped collard or greens of your choice.

Brown rice or other rice that is higher in fiber may require more water as not only do they need to be cooked for longer but they will also absorb more water. I recommend 125ml water to 100g rice or, if using cups, 1 and 1/4 cups to 1 cup rice. Bring to a rolling boil and then reduce the heat to a gentle simmer. Cook for 30 mins then turn off the heat. Quickly cover with a lid and leave tightly covered for another 5-10 mins to absorb any remaining water.

Meanwhile, in a non-stick pan, heat the beet broth, saute the onion until soften. Set aside.
Place the garlic in a clean non-stick pan, add the balsamic and water, on medium heat, saute both side until soften and get brown color. Set aside.

Add the sauted onion, salt and black pepper in the rice, stir well to combine together. Divide between plates. Top with sauted garlic, celeriac crumb and fresh dill.

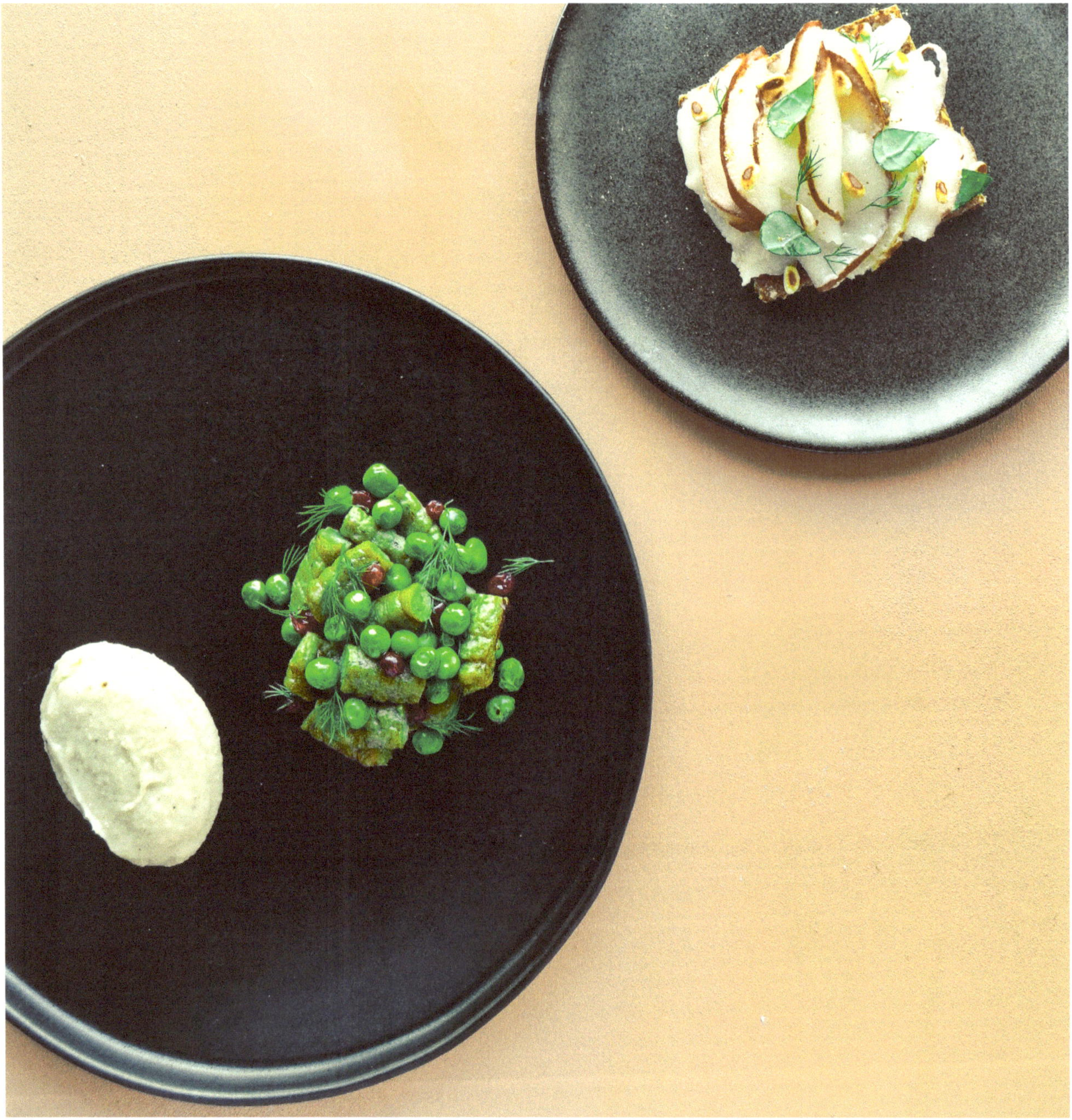

KOHLRABI GNOCCHI WITH COLLARD

A kind of experimental dish turned into a festival. Gnocchi made of root vegetables are both nutritious and delicious. You can also pair it with tomato sauce or yogurt.

Time - 40 minutes
Serves - 4

1 large kohlrabi (365 g measured after tops and skin removed)
60 g fresh collard greens
165 g buckwheat flour + more as needed for kneading
55 g tapioca flour + 4 tbsp water
1 tbsp psyllium powder
Salt and pepper to taste
2 tbsp balsamic
Roasted celeriac oat puree to serve (page 143)

Garnish
Cracked black pepper
2 springs green onions
2 tbsp fresh dill
1/4 toasted green peas fresh or defrosted
1 tbsp capers (optional)
1 tbsp lingon jam (optional)

Peel and cut the kohlrabi, cook in boiling water until soft. The smaller you cut it, the shorter the boiling time is. I found that for 1-inch cubes it takes approx. 8-10 minutes.
In a small food processor, puree the collard with a little bit water 1 tbsp at one time.
Smash the kohlrabi with a fork and use your hand to combine it with collard puree, buckwheat flour, tapioca, psyllium, water, salt, and pepper. Don't overwork it.

Take a small piece and form long tubes. Keep a good amount of buckwheat flour close by when you're rolling and cutting your gnocchi – depending on the moisture level of your kohlrabi, you may need a sprinkling of it from time to time. Then cut the tubes into inch-long pieces. You can add stripes to your gnocchi by pushing them against a fork.

Cook your gnocchi in boiling water. It takes about 1 minute for the gnocchi pieces to rise to the surface. Wait another 2 minutes and you can take them out with a strainer. They will get plenty of time to cook in the pan, so just a couple minutes in boiling water is enough. If you let them get too soft they risk falling apart.

Heat the balsamic in a large frying pan over a medium heat. then add the gnocchi. Cook for 3 mins until starting to brown, add the green peas and cook for 2-3 minutes by stirring constantly. Once done, toss with green onions, fresh dill, capers, lingon jam and sprinkle some black pepper. Serve along with roasted celeriac puree! (page 143)

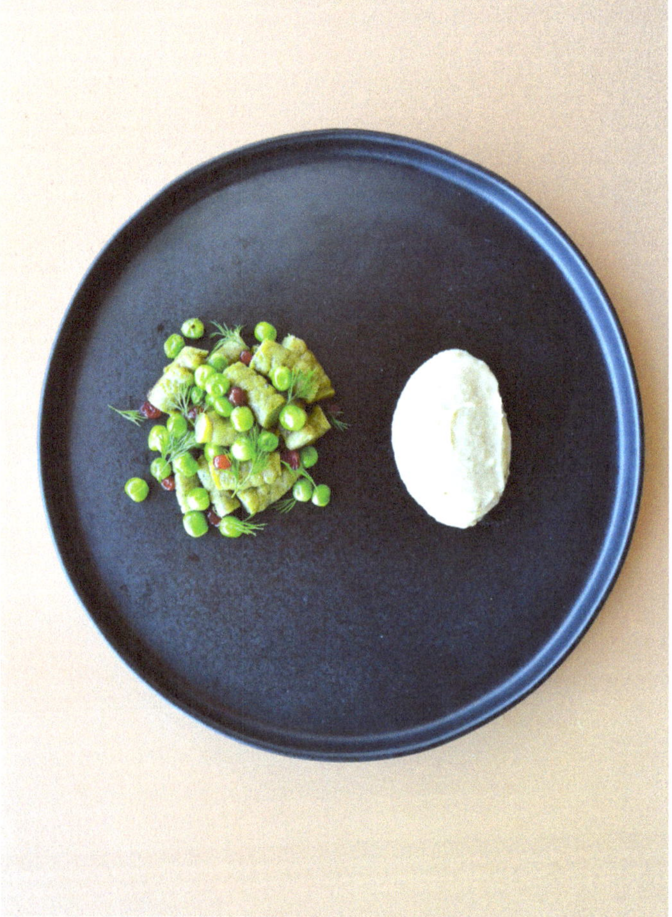

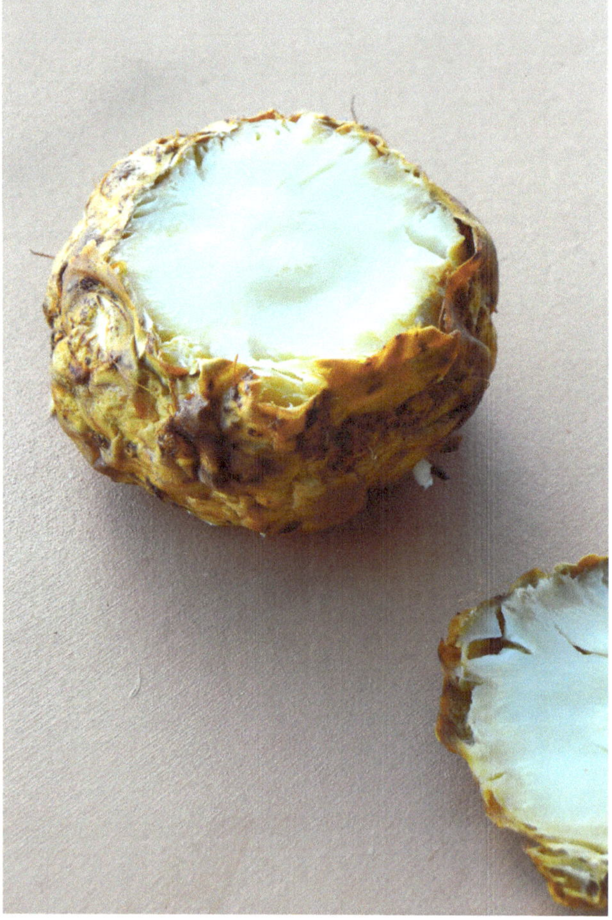

ROASTED OAT CELERIAC PUREE

Creamy rich almost like white chocolate cream celeriac purée can me make easily without oil. You can boil it and blend with the water in the blender of course, but with the roasting, all the flavours keep inside and caramelising boost the flavour of celeriac. Turning simple ingredient like celery root into something is outstanding!

Time - 2 hours roastings + 10 min prep
Serves - 4

50 g celeriac (measured after tops and skin peeled and cubed)
1 tbsp vegetable broth or balsamic
240 ml oat milk (or 2 tbsp gluten-free rolled oats + 240 ml water)
1/4 tsp salt
Freshly ground black pepper to taste

Preheat oven to 180º C.
Line a baking tray with parchment paper.

Cut the tops aways, peel the skin of the celeriac and then cut your celeriac into small cubes. Massage with veg broth or balsamic and salt. Transfer to baking tray.
Bake in the oven until soft and golden.

Once it is done, remove from the oven, transfer to a high speed blender. Add the oat milk. (Never add too much liquid once.) Blend until smooth. If you need more liquid to reach the desired consistency, add only one tablespoon at a time.

Taste, adjust the pepper and salt.

Strain through a fine sieve. Serve with your gnocchi. This sauce is also great to serve with vegetable meatballs, falafel etc.

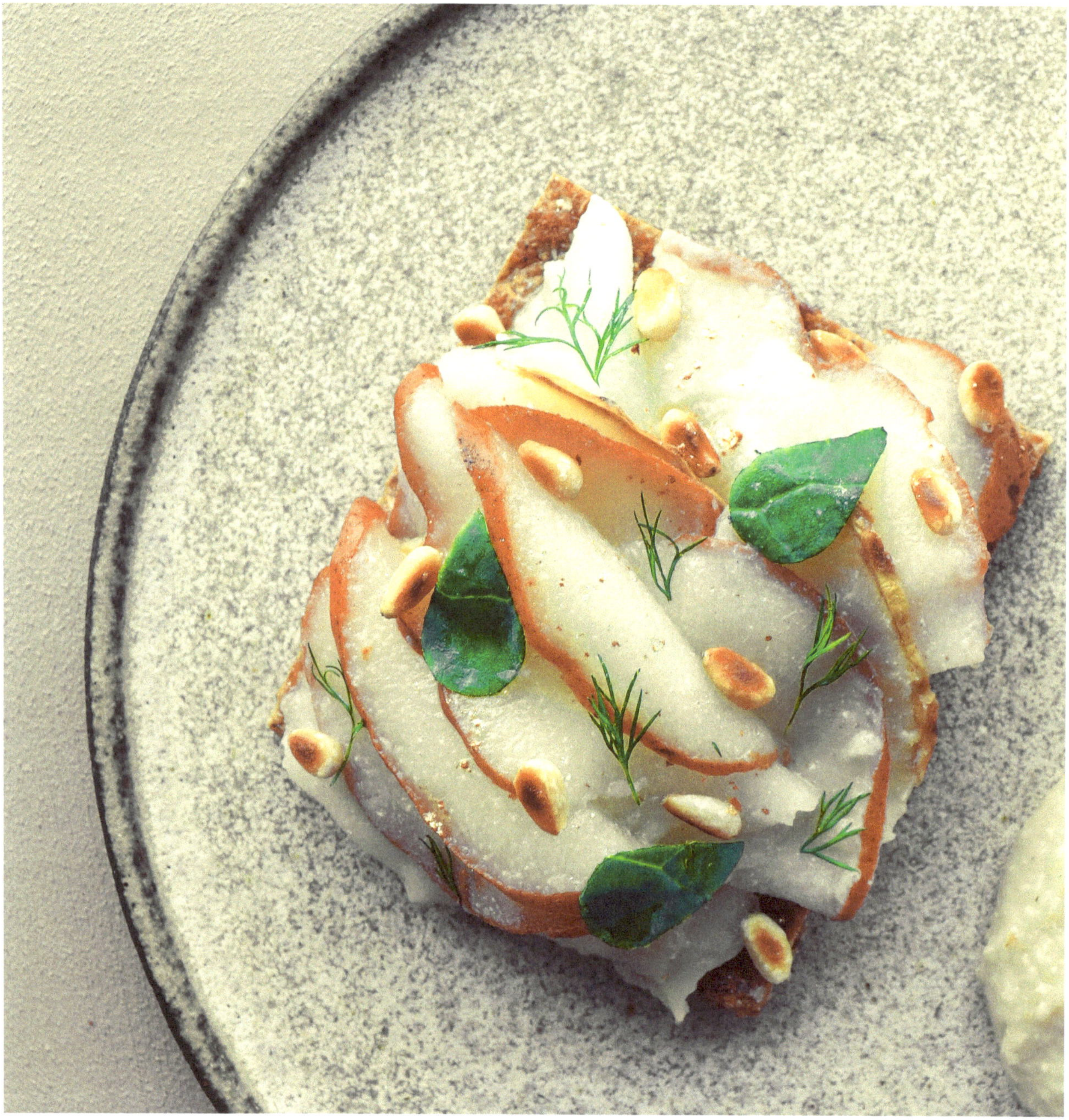

ROASTED CELERIAC AND PEAR WITH MUSTARD DRESSING

This festive dish can be served as a starter, sharing dish or a main on the buckwheat or cauliflower bread. Also perfect on the top of farinata.

Time - 2 hours roastings + 10 min prep
Serves - 4

2 head celeriac
1 large santa maria pear
1 tsp balsamic
1 tsp salt
1 tbsp toasted pine nuts
1 tsp pickled capers
1 tbsp fresh dill
Collard green cut into small leaves (optional)

Mustard Dressing
1 tsp dijon mustard
1 tsp seaweed blend (nori,wakame,dulse)
2 tbsp lemon juice
1 tbsp water to thin

Preheat oven to 175° C.
Cut the leaves of the celeriac, remove and keep in the refrigerator. You can use them in another recipe.
Wash and rub the celeriac with salt. Do not peel them, we will bake with their skin. Just make sure your celeriac is relatively clean.
Wash and drain a large santa maria pear.
Place the celeriacs and pear on the oven wire mesh, roast in the lower middle part of the oven.
Check on the celeriac and turn it around every 30 minutes.
After 2 hours it will be ready. It should be soft all the way through, if it is not, continue to cook another 30 minutes or as needed. When your celeriac is done, it should look slightly dehydrated but not burn after that time in the oven (see picture on page 142).
Blend the dressing ingredients in a bowl or blender and set aside.
Arrange the rest of the ingredients while roasting the celeriac.
Wash and drain your dill, toast pine nuts, drain capers.
Once celeriac and pear roasted, let them cool for 10 minutes, then using a mandolin slicer, thinly slice. Cut away to top and buttom. You may also want to carve the skin before slicing, othewise it is totally good to consume it with its skin.
Toss with mustard dressing, add the balsamic, capers, dill, collard, and pine nuts. This dish can be served immediately at room temperature, also good cold if you want to make beforehand and serve the next day.

OAT PUMPKIN RISOTTO WITH SAMPHIRE, QUINCE AND POMEGRANATES

Time - 1 hour 45 minutes

Serves - 2 person

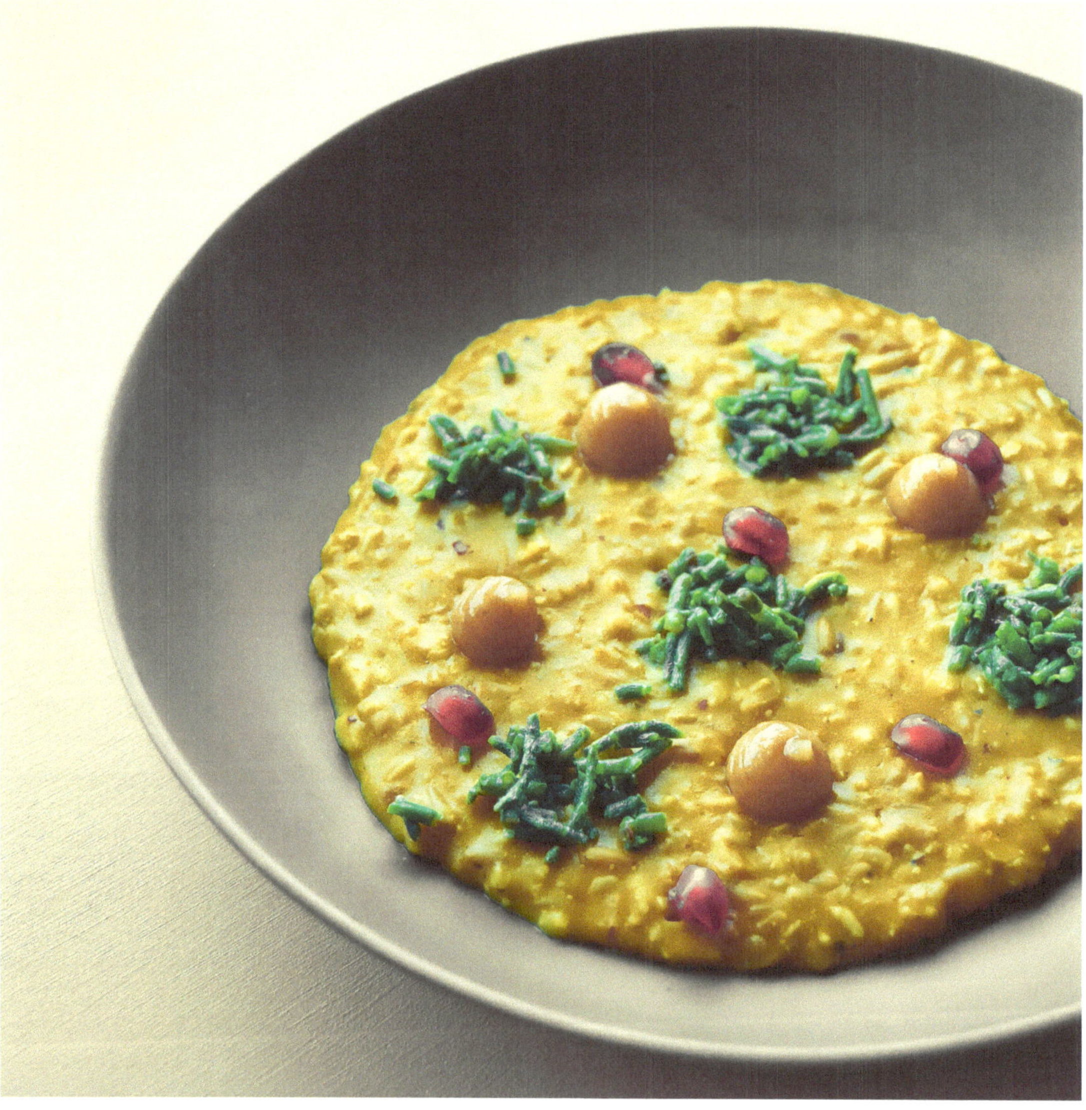

Oat Risotto

500 g pumpkin cubed
1 large red onion finelly chopped
3 garlic cloves minced
1/4 cup beetroot broth
1 bay leaf
1/4 tsp cayenne
150 g whole oats (or steel cut)
1 cup filtered water
Salt and pepper to taste
1/4 cup pomegranates to serve

Quince Puree

2 ripe quinces
40 g date puree
1/2 tsp cardamom
1 star anise
1 cinnamon stick
1 clove
1 tbsp lemon juice
2 cups water
A pinch salt

Sauted Samphire

1/2 bunch samphire
1/4 cup white vegetable broth

TIPS - Whole and steel cut oats are the texture of a grain like rice or barley, so they require much more cooking than rolled oats. You can soak them beforehand to reduce the cooking time.

Place whole or steel cut oats in a bowl, wash and dry. Cover with water, let it sit overnight or for 10-12 hours.
Then strain the excess water. Cook for 20 - 25 minutes.
Peel and cut your pumpkins, cut into cubes. Place in a deep pot, cover with water. Add a whole bay leaf. Bring to a simmer over high heat, then reduce heat to medium and simmer for 20 mins or until the pumpkin is very tender. Strain and set aside to cool them.
In a skillet, saute the onions and garlic in the beetroot broth. Once soften, transfer to a blender, then add the pumpkins and 1-2 tbsp water as needed to make it puree.
Pour the pumpkin puree over the cooked oats. Stir well and continue to cook in the pumpkin puree for 10-12 minutes or until oats absorbs the water content and tender. Serve your risotto with quince puree drops, sauted samphire and pomegranate seeds for a gourmet effect. Alternatively you can serve as it is or with pepper and nut parmesan.

To make quince puree, peel the quince, remove the core, then cut into quarters. Place in a pot, cover with 2 cups water. Add the star anise, clove, cinnamon stick and cardamom. Cook the quinces on low-medium temperature (simmer) for about 45-50 minutes, depending on how tough and big the fruits are. Once done, drain and transfer fruits in a high speed blender, add the another date puree, a pinch salt and lemon juice. Blend until smooth puree.

To prepare the samphire, rinse the samphire thoroughly and trim off any tough ends. If you have large clumps then break them up a bit. Place them in a large skillet, add the vegetable broth or water, cook on high heat until absorbs the water and tender for about 2-3 minutes.

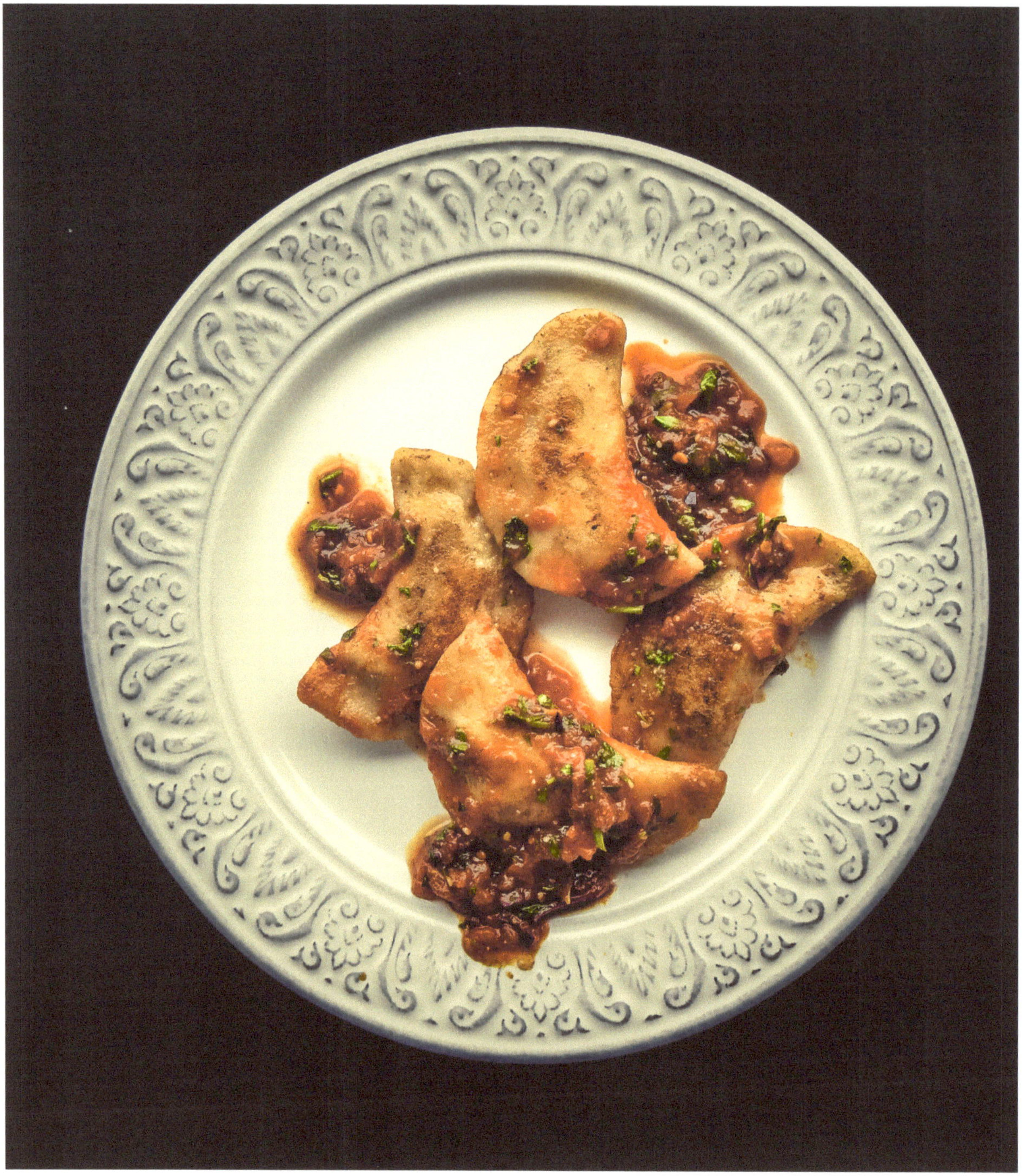

MUSHROOM PIEROGI

Time - 40 minutes

Serves - 4 person

Dough

90 g buckwheat flour

70 g brown rice flour

60 g cassava or tapioca

1 tbsp psyllium powder

1/2 tsp salt

180 ml water

Filling

400 g mushrooms chopped

2 red onion chopped

A handful of greens (kale, spinach, collard etc.)

1 large red bell pepper chopped

60 ml vegetable broth

4 garlic cloves minced

1 tsp salt

1/2 tsp ground bay leaf

1/2 tsp chili flakes

1/4 tsp blackpepper

Sauce

400 g shredded tomatoes

2 tbsp tomato paste

1/4 bunch chopped parsley

4 garlic cloves minced

1 tbsp balsamic

Salt and pepper to taste

To prepare the filling, place the chopped onion, garlic, pepper and mushrooms in a non-stick skillet, add the vegetable broth and ground bay leaf. Gently cook until translucent and lightly caramelised. Once done, add the chili, black pepper and salt. Lastly add the chopped greens, toss together and set aside.

In a large-bottomed bowl, whisk together the buckwheat flour, brown rice flour, cassava, psyllium and salt. Then add the water. Gradually begin stirring the flour mixture with the water in the center. The dough should hold together without being overly wet and sticky. If it is too dry, add 1-2 tbsp water. If it is too wet, add some buckwheat flour until archieve the desired texture.

Prepare a clean counter or pastry mat by dusting with buckwheat flour. Divide the dough in half, turning one half of the dough onto the dusted surface. Begin rolling the dough by rolling gently in one direction, then in the other, to form a 1/8 inch thick round of dough.

Cut out circle shapes for individual pierogies using a large glass or round cutter (7 cm / 2.75"). Place a teaspoon of the filling in the middle of each circle, and then fold the circle over the dough so it forms a half-moon shaped pocket. Pinch the edges together firmly. Dip your finger in water to dab around the edge if needed. The dough is much less stretchy than normal dough so take care to not overfill.

Keep finished pierogies on a baking sheet. When ready to serve, boil pierogies for 5-6 minutes, stirring very gently. Once they begin to float, drain pierogies and toss with balsamic or vegetable broth, and serve with tomato parsley sauce and nut topping if desired.

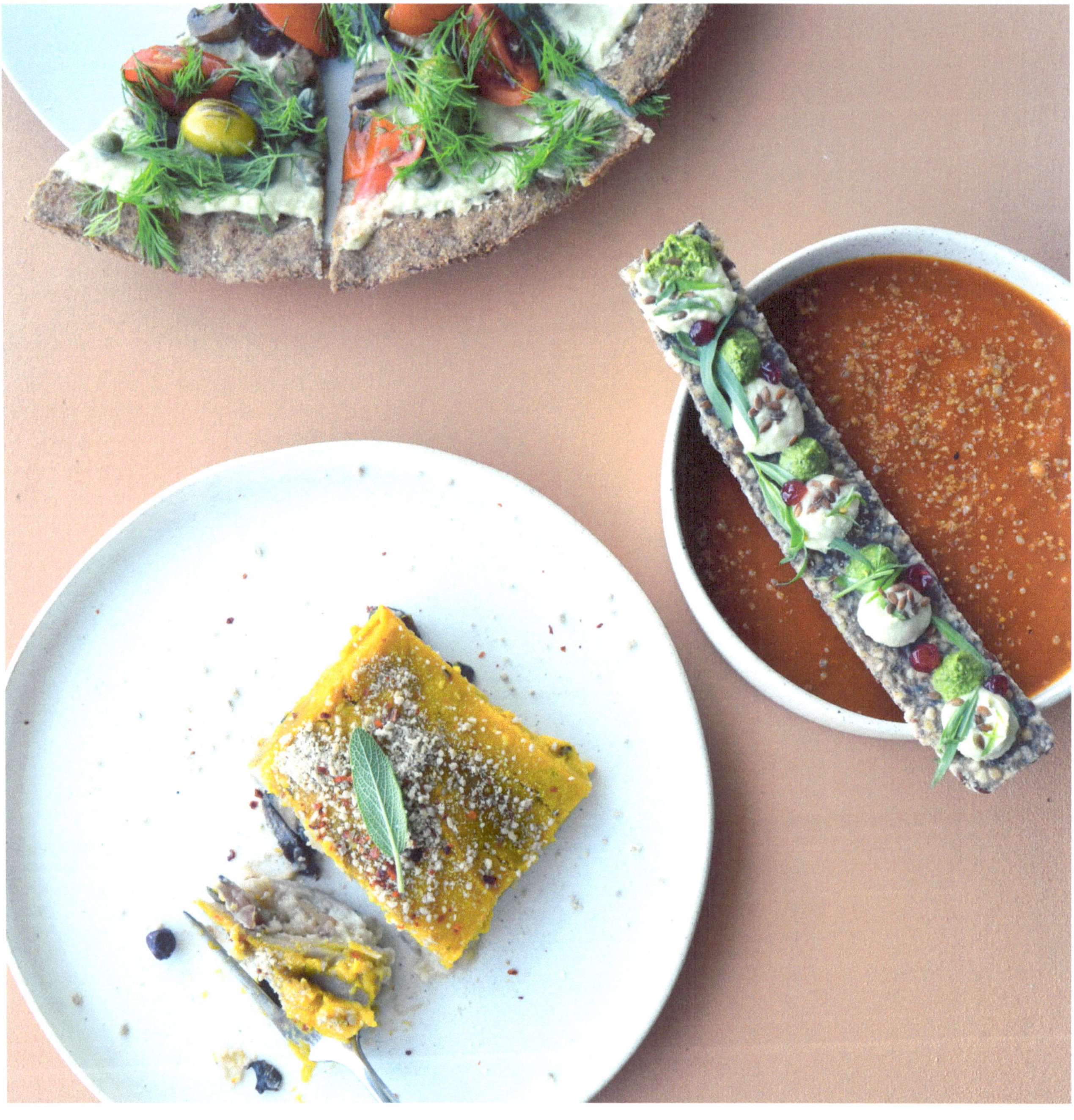

BUCKWHEAT LASAGNA WITH MUSHROOMS CAULIFLOWER BECHAMEL AND PUMPKIN CHEDDAR

Time - 80 minutes

Serves - 4 person

Dough

1 and 1/4 cup buckwheat flour

1/2 cup cassava or tapioca flour

2 tbsp psyllium husk powder

150 ml water

1/4 tsp salt

Cauliflower Bechamel

400 g cauliflower florets

1 sweet onion chopped

120 ml almond milk as needed for creamy consistency (start with less)

Generous pinch of salt as needed

1/8 tsp cayenne

A pinch ground nutmeg

1 bay leaf

To serve

1/2 cup nut parmesan (mixture of 1/4 cup sunflower seeds, 1/2 tsp garlic powder, 1/4 salt and 1/4 orange peel powder)

1 cup fresh baby spinach leaves, cherry tomatoes tossed with 1 tbsp balsamic

Mushroom Filling

1 red onion finely chopped

4 garlic cloves minced

300 g mushroom chopped (cremini, button, shiitake, portobello, wild mushrooms, etc.)

4 tbsp beetroot broth

1/4 tsp salt

1/4 tsp ground black pepper

1 cup spinach, kale or collard (optional)

Butternut Squash Cheddar

400 g butternut squash chopped

1 red onion chopped

2 garlic cloves minced

1/4 tsp ground mustard

4 tbsp vegetable broth

1/4 cup water

1/2 tsp salt

1/2 tsp red pepper flakes

1 tbsp sage

lasagna continued

Lasagna Dough

In a bowl, whisk together the flour, tapioca, and salt until well-combined.

Add the psyllium, water and start with the first 6 tbsp of water. Mix with a wooden spoon until a nice dough forms. You are looking for slightly moist but not sticky at all.

If your dough is still too dry, add the remaining tablespoons of water. At some point you are going to have to ditch the wooden spoon and start using your hands so you can feel the consistency and knead the dough. If it's too sticky add a tablespoon of buckwheat flour until moist but not sticky.

Remove dough from the bowl, place on to your buckwheat floured surface.
Once the dough is silky and smooth, you can begin to roll it out more thinly. Roll it once through each of the next two or three settings, adding flour as needed, until the dough is about 1/4-inch thick. Once the pasta is about 1/4-inch thick, begin rolling it twice through the next thinner settings.

The rectangle lasagne pieces are generally cut to approximately 3 ½ x 5 inches or 4 x 6 inches, using a knife to create a straight edge.
When deciding on what size to use, consider the size of the baking dish that you will be using and use a size that will work best for the dish. Sprinkle with more buckwheat flour to prevent sticking together.

Butternut Squash Cheddar Sauce

Preheat oven to 200° C.

Cut butternut squash in half, scoop out the seeds and place open side down on a parchment-lined baking sheet.

Place sliced onion next to it and drizzle it with 2 tbsp vegetable broth.

Roast until fork-tender, about 30-40 minutes. Let cool. You could do this a day before or cook whole in an instant pot for 22 minutes.

In a large pan, saute the onions and garlic in 3 tbsp vegetable broth until soften.

When the butternut squash is cool enough to handle, scoop all the flesh out into a food processor. Add the sauted onion and garlic along with the water, mustard, sage, salt, pepper. Puree until smooth.

Cauliflower Bechamel

Cauliflower is one of winter's wonders. In her ruffled white coat, she is both delicate and creamy with a gentle bite of her coniferous vegetable heritage and while the world thinks cauliflower needs to become pizza crust, or gnocchi, or a smoothie base, I think we can also celebrate as a bechamel.

Add the cauliflower to a large pot and add water to cover. Bring to a boil medium high heat and cook until the cauliflower is very tender, about 10 minutes.

Drain the excess water and puree the cauliflower using an immersion blender or in a blender with a tight-fitting lid.

Place the onion and garlic along with 2 tbsp vegetable broth in a large skillet or saucepan and saute over medium heat for 5-6 minutes.

Add the cooked onion and garlic and rest of the ingredients in the blender, mix with the cauliflower, add more almond milk if needed, to achieve a creamy consistency. Blend until smooth.

Mushroom Filling

In a large skillet, heat the beetroot broth.

Add chopped onions and garlic in the skillet. Saute the onion and garlic first for 2 minutes stirring often.

Then add the mushrooms and cook on medium heat another 7 minutes or until the mushrooms release their liquid and begin to brown.

Stir 1-2 more times, leaving mushrooms alone for a couple of minutes in between. Once there is almost no moisture left in the skillet, and the mushrooms are a deeply browned color,turn the heat off.

You could toss in some spinach, kale or collard at the end and wilt for extra nutrients.

To wilt greens, just toss with the mushrooms, they will become soft and bright green in couple of seconds.

Taste and make sure the filling has enough salt and pepper. You could make this the day ahead and refrigerate.

TIPS

Do not wash your mushrooms. Once wet, mushrooms are nearly impossible to fully dry, which makes it less likely they'll take on that golden color and those crispy edges when you sauté them. Worse still, if you wash and then store mushrooms in a sealed container, they'll start to turn slimy before they even meet your your lasagna.

However, you should still clean your mushrooms before you start cooking. Dry-cleaning method is to take a dry vegetable brush or crumpled paper towel to brush away any clods of dirt or other debris clinging to food. Cultivated mushrooms such as supermarket buttons and cremini are generally grown in sterilized compost, so chances are anything clinging to these will be fairly inert and hardly noticeable after cooking. And it's definitely not going to make you sick, which is the most important thing.

Foraged mushrooms like chanterelles, morels, and black trumpets often have pine needles and other debris stuck to them, which makes some degree of cleaning necessary, but the dry-cleaning method above will work just fine.

Assemble

In a 9 x13 inch baking dish, add 1 cup of the butternut puree and spread out into a thin layer.

Top with lasagna sheets.

Spread 1/2 of the bechamel sauce. Top with half of the sauted mushrooms and spread evently. Sprinkle with 1/4 cup nut parmesan.

Add more lasagna sheets.

Spoon half of the remaining butternut puree, erring on the side of less than half, so you have enough to cover the top (save at least 1 ¼ cups for the top.)

Add the remaining mushrooms and all the good bits and sprinkle with another ½ cup nut parmesan. Pour the rest of the bechamel over the mushrooms.

Place the final sheets over the top. Lather with the remaining butternut puree and sprinkle with the rest of the nut parmesan. You could assemble this 1-2 days before baking.

Bake in 190° C oven for 40 minutes.

After 40 minutes, check it, add 1/4 cup almond milk over the lasagna if it looks so dry and continue baking 15-20 minutes until golden and bubbly. Cut into slices and serve with chopped sage leaves.

TIPS

Without resting, lasagna turns into a molten mess. So we can say that letting the lasagna rest is key to successful serving. You need to wait at least 10 minutes, and up to 20 if you can stand it, before cutting into your lasagna.Giving it this time will allow it to set up and ensure that each square holds its shape.

MAKING GLUTEN-FREE BREAD CRUMBS FROM SCRATCH

Time - 25 minutes

1 small buckwheat bread loaf (page 59)
Salt and spices

Place the buckwheat bread onto a cutting board.
Cut it into 1-inch cubes.
Add the bread cubes to a food processor.
Process until you get fine. It's okay if you have a smaller food processor, just process in batches.
Spread the gluten-free bread crumbs onto a parchment lined baking sheet. I like using parchment paper , it's easier to transfer the breadcrumbs to a container.

Bake at 190° C until gets golden brown. If desired, once the breadcrumbs have cooled, add seasonings.

Storage
Place completely cooled breadcrumbs in a glass container or a zip lock bag in a cool, dry place. If you aren't going to use them within a month or so, place them in the freezer.

If you store them in the freezer make sure you bring them to room temperature before you use them.

TIPS
You can also use almond meal instead of buckwheat bread, almond meal has a coarse texture and a nutty flavor, making it a great gluten-free substitute for bread crumbs.

KATSU CURRY

Time - 35 minutes
Serves - 4

2 large aubergine
1 sweet potato
1/2 cup cassava or tapioca
1 cup oat milk
100 g breadcrumbs (page 156)
2 tbsp sesame seeds

For the Curry Sauce
1 tbsp sunflower seed butter
1 large red onion finely diced
4 garlic cloves diced
3 tsp finely grated ginger
2 medium carrots peeled sliced
1/2 granny smith apple peeled diced
3 tbsp mushroom stock or tamari
3 tsp curry powder
1 tbsp mirin or maple syrup
1/2 tsp salt

To Serve
Cooked brown rice
Chopped lettuce or greens

Heat up 2 tbsp beetroot broth in a pan. Add diced onion and sauté until almost transparent, add garlic and a minute or two later add ginger. Fry for another minute or two stirring frequently. Add sliced carrot, diced apple and curry powder. Stir around and fry off for a minute or two. Simmer, on low heat (with a lid on) for about 10-15 minutes until carrots and apples become soft. Transfer to an upright blender or use a stick blender to make a smooth, thick sauce. Season with mushroom stock or tamari and maple or mirin. Add more water if the sauce is too thick.

Prepare 4 plates. Pour about ½ cup of breadcrumb on the first one. Season the cassava with generous amount of salt and pepper. Pour the oat milk onto the second plate. Pour breadcrumbs and a handful of white sesame seeds onto the third plate and line the fourth plate with double layer of paper towel.

Cut aubergine and sweet potato into ½ cm or 0.2 inch thick slices. Don't make them thicker.

Dip the slices in seasoned cassava first, then in oat milk and finally in breadcrumbs. Press the breadcrumbs into the slices and shake each piece gently before putting onto hot oil to allow excess bread-crumbs to come off.

Bake in the preheated oven at 200° C until the coating becomes golden brown.

Serve with brown rice, a simple green salad and a generous amount of curry sauce.

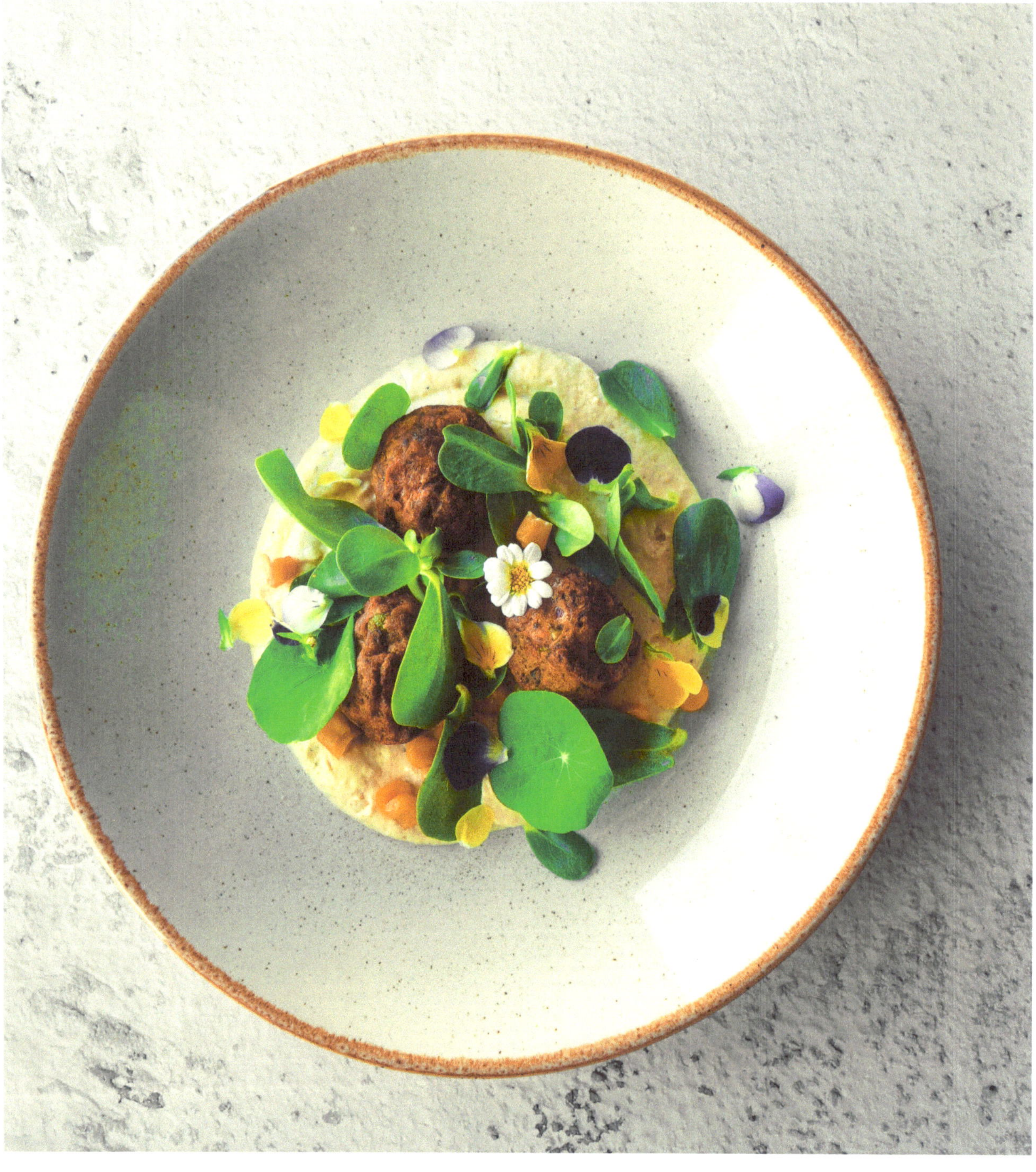

VEGBALLS WITH SUNFLOWER SEED CREAM AND PURSLANE

Time - 45 minutes
Serves - 2 person

1/2 cup brown basmati rice + 1.5 cup water
2 tbsp balsamic + 2 tbsp water
60 g thinly sliced red onion
3 garlic cloves minced
250 g sliced button mushrooms
105 g sunflower seeds
90 g gluten-free oat flour
1/2 tsp sea salt
1/4 tsp chili pepper
1/4 tsp ground black pepper
2 tbsp mushroom stock (tamari or coconut aminos)

Sunflower Seed Cream
90 g sunflower seeds soaked in warm water for 30 min.
4-5 tbsp water
3 tbsp lemon juice
2 tbsp nutritional yeast
1/4 tsp blackpepper
1/4 tsp pink himalayan salt

Wash and rinse your brown rice, place in a pot, cover with 1.5 cup water. Cook until the rice absorbs all the water content and soften. Once your rice cooked it should be around 205 grams. Let it cool at least 15-20 minutes.

Place 1 tbsp balsamic in a skillet, add the sliced onions and garlic. Sauté on medium heat until onions begin to turn golden, then turn the heat down to low. Add the 2 tbsp water to prevent burning and cook for 1-2 minutes stirring constantly.

Then add the chopped mushrooms, another 1 tbsp balsamic and 2 tbsp mushroom stock. Sauté for about 5 minutes, stirring regularly, until the mushrooms are fragrant and soft. Once done, remove from the stove, let it cool for 10 minutes.

Meanwhile add the sunflower seeds in a food processor, pulse until crumb texture. Remove from the food processor, set aside.

Add the cooled rice to your empty food processor and pulse until slightly crumbled.

Then add the cooked mushrooms, garlic and onions and pulse until well combined.

Now add the oat flour, start with lesser amounts and add more as needed.

Vegballs continued

Add the 1 tbsp tamari, salt, chili and black pepper. Pulse for 2-3 times.
Lastly add the sunflower seed crumb and pulse twice.
The texture should be thick and sticky, also easy to form into patties. If it is too wet, add more oat flour and stir by hand. Taste and adjust the salt and pepper if needed.
Make small balls from the dough. Cook on the skillet at medium-high temperature with little bit balsamic, tamari or beetroot broth for about 4-5 minutes until golden and crispy.
To make sunflower seed cream, place all sunflower seed cream ingredients in the blendec twister jar. Mix on high speed until you get smooth silky cream.
To serve, pour 2-3 tbsp cream to the middle of the plate.
Place some purslane over the sauce.
Put 2-3 vegetable balls to the plate. Add the corns.
Decorate with fresh dill and edible flowers.

This dish also can be served with the basic tomato sauce instead of sunflower seed cream. If you want to try this way, recipe is given below.

BASIC TOMATO SAUCE

Time - 10 min prep + 25 min baking
Makes around 1 litre / 4 cups

2 tbsp beetroot broth
1 yellow onion, finely chopped
2 garlic cloves, finely chopped
1/2 tsp dried chili
3 x 400 g cans whole plum tomatoes
5 sprigs of basil, leaves picked
sea salt and freshly ground pepper

Heat oil in a saucepan on medium heat. Add onion, garlic and chili and sauté for a couple of minutes until golden. Stir in the tomatoes, basil, salt and pepper. Use a wooden spoon to crush the tomatoes. Lower the heat, cover and gently simmer for about 20 minutes. Use immediately or cool and store in an air-tight glass jar in the fridge. Keeps for about a week.

SPAGHETTI SQUASH WITH TOMATO SAUCE

Time - 10 min prep + 40 min baking
Serves - 2-3 person

1 kg spaghetti squash
1 tbsp beetroot broth
Sea salt
Freshly ground black pepper

To Serve
Basic tomato sauce (page 160)

Spaghetti squash is a nutritious winter vegetable that offers lots of fiber, beta-carotene, folate and more. It offers a really fun, spaghetti-like texture and built-in bowl shape.

Preheat the oven to 200° C.
Slice the spaghetti squash in half lengthwise or four pieces and scoop out the seeds and ribbing.
Massage the inside of the squash with beet broth and sprinkle with salt and pepper.

Place the spaghetti squash cut side down on the baking sheet and use a fork to poke holes. Roast for 40 minutes or until lightly browned on the outside, fork tender, but still a litte bit firm. Do not bake too much otherwise you will end with a squash puree!

Remove from the oven and flip the squash so that it's cut side up.
When cool to the touch, use a fork to scrape and fluff the strands from the sides of the squash.

One of the best ways to eat spaghetti squash is to combine with basic tomato sauce. It is also great when combined with spicy chickpeas. Mushroom, kale and plant-based parmesan combo is also great!

"DESSERTS ARE EDIBLE LOVE"

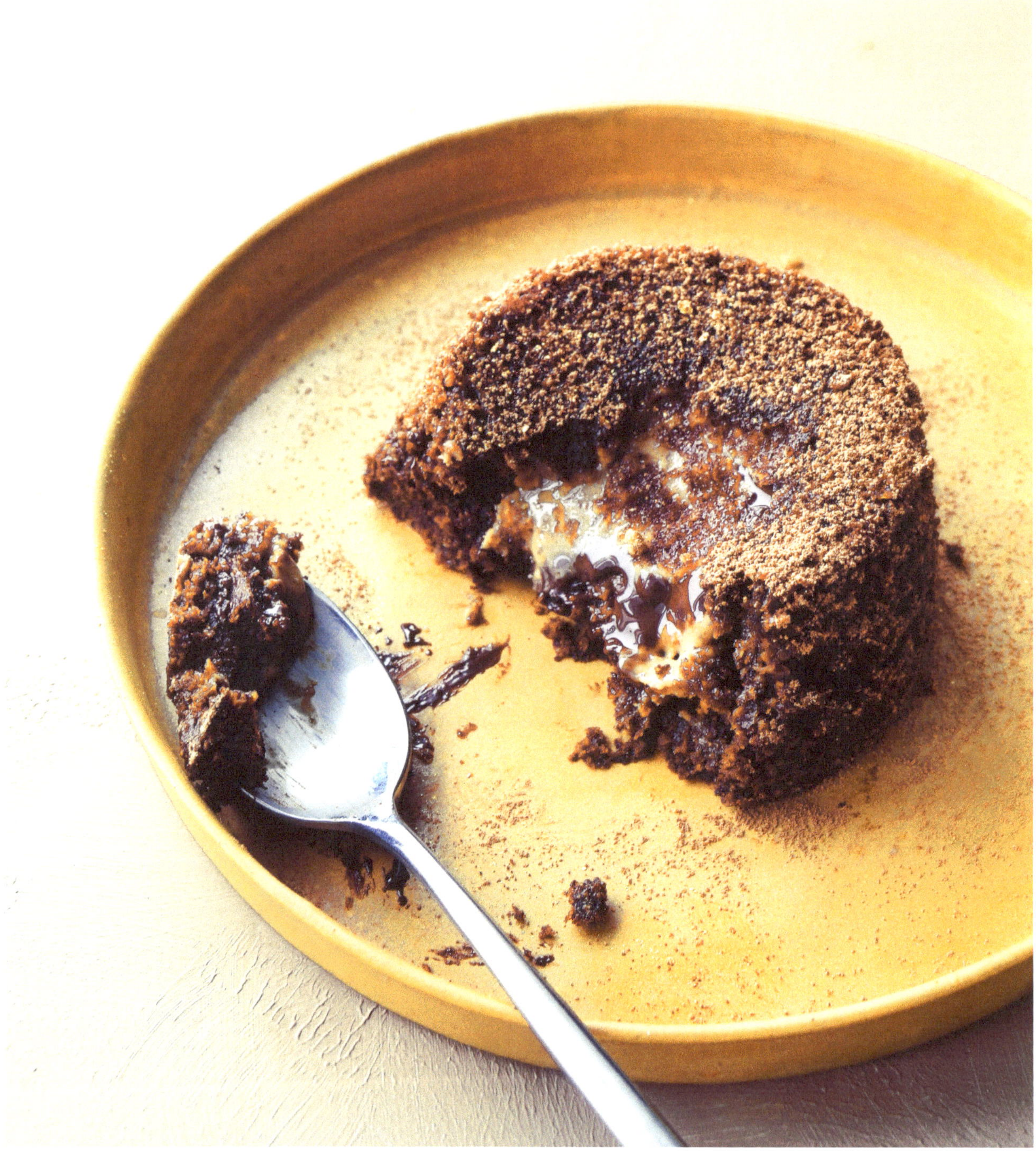

LAVA CAKE

This delicious lava cake with a gooey center is super simple and makes 2 individual chocolate lava cakes. Use carob instead of cacao or cherry jam in the place of chocolate if you have any issue with the chocolate or cacao.

Time - 7 min prep + 18 min baking
Serves - 2 person

50 g cup oat flour
40 g date paste
15 g cacao powder or carob
1/2 tsp baking powder
60 g banana
80 g oat milk
25 g almond butter
1/4 tsp apple cider vinegar

Filling
1/2 tbsp almond butter
1 square gluten-free vegan chocolate or cherry jam

Preheat the oven to 180° C.
Mix the oat flour, cacao powder and baking powder together.

In another bowl, mash the banana with a fork. Then add the almond butter and date paste.
Add the oat milk and apple cider vinegar then mix well.

Pour some half of the batter into each soufflé mold (about 3 inches in diameter, use the silicon one, otherwise you may need to grease the molds.)

Add the almond butter and a piece of chocolate on top.
Cover with the rest of the batter.

Bake for 18 minutes. Once baked, remove the mold by inverting it onto the plate.
Dust some cacao on top. Serve immediately!

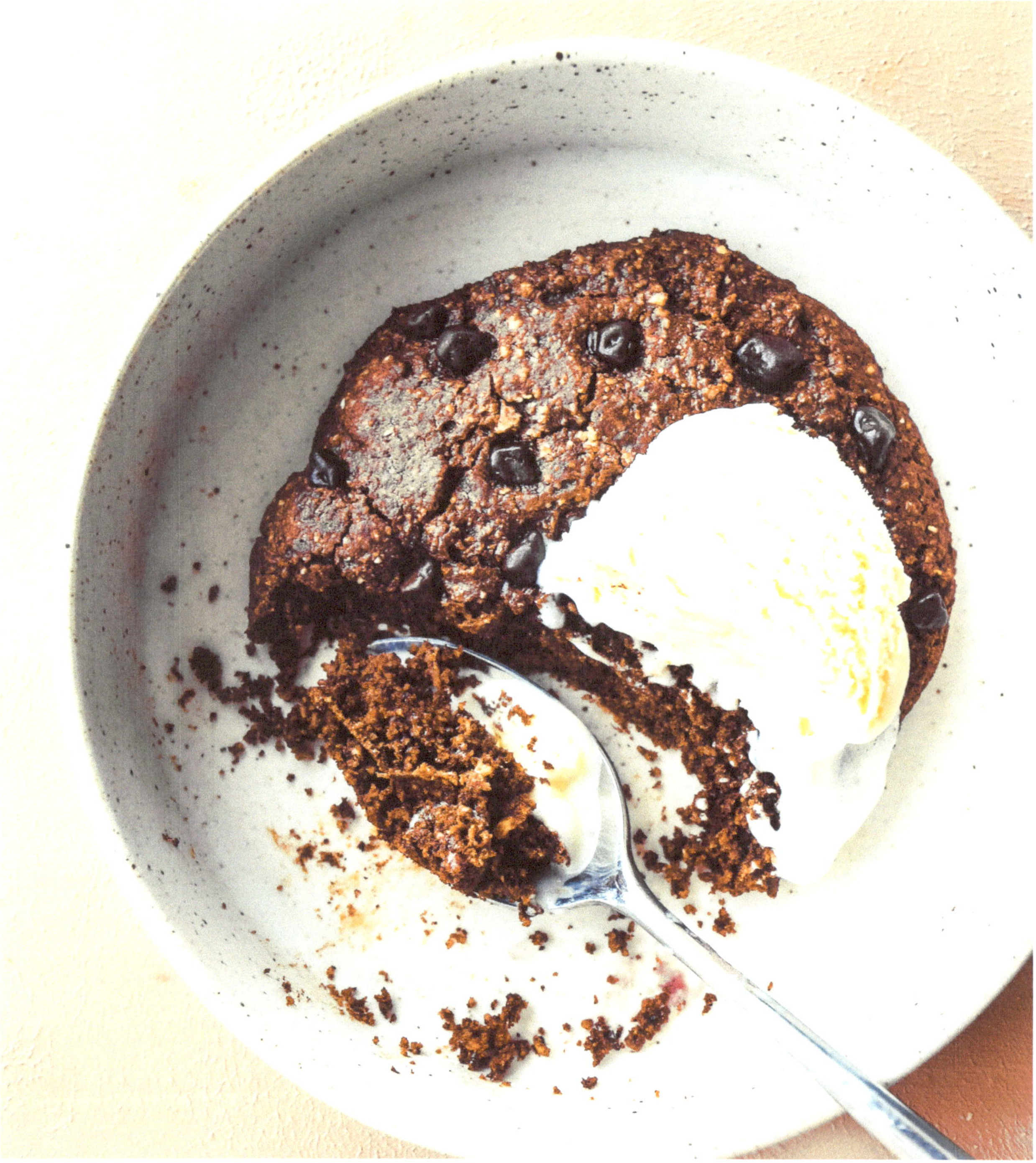

GIANT COOKIE CAKE

This giant cookie is perfect for breakfast, a snack, or a treat!

Time - 8 min prep + 12 min baking
Serves - 1 giant cookie

1 tsp chia seeds + 2 tbsp water
65 g walnut flour
2 tbsp cacao or carob
1 tbsp date paste
2 tbsp maple syrup
3 tbsp hazelnut butter
1/4 tsp salt
1/4 tsp baking powder
2 tbsp chocolate chips (optional if you are using chocolate, or add dried cherries)

TIPS

If you don't consume chocolate, make this recipe with cinnamon (1 tsp) and dried raisins (1/4 cup).

Preheat oven to 175° C.

In a bowl, mix chia seeds and water. Keep stirring for the first minute or so to prevent the chia seeds from clumping together. Then set aside for 5 minutes.

Then add all the rest of the ingredients over the chia seeds. Stir well to combine.

Fold in the chopped chocolate (save a few pieces for garnish).

Transfer the dough onto a baking tray lined parchment paper. Lightly wet your hands and shape the dough into a large cookie, about 1 inch thick. The cookie won't spread that much, so shape it the way you want the end result to look like. Top with the remaining chocolate.

Bake in the middle of the oven for 12 minutes, or until cracks begin to form. The cookie won't get that much color, so take it out and trust that it is done. We don't want to over-bake it. Let it sit for 30 minutes to cool and settle.

Once it is somewhat cool the cookie is ready to broken into pieces and served! If you like to eat warm cookie, eat with a scoop of vanilla ice cream on top.

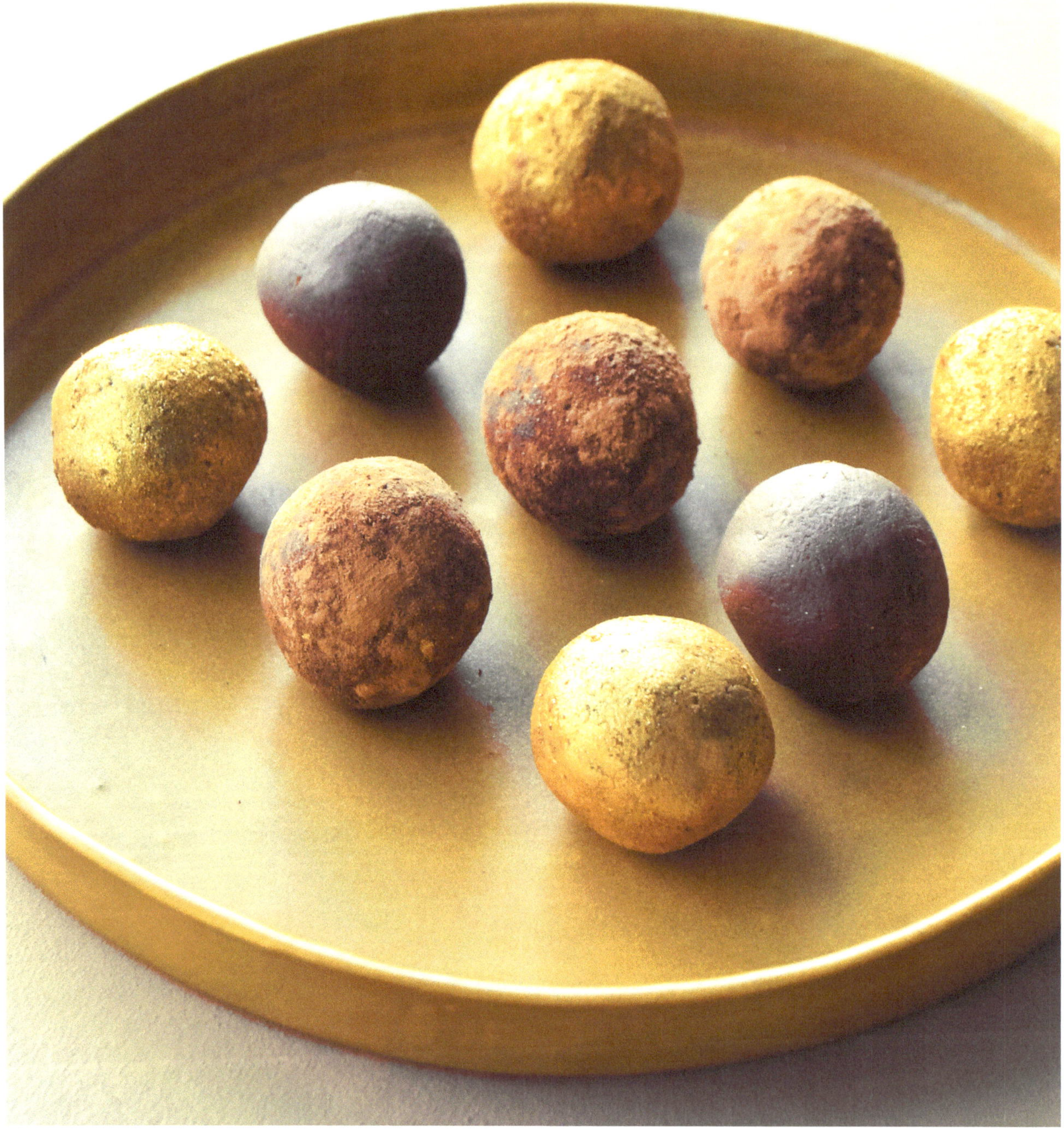

CHESTNUT CHOCOLATE TRUFFLES

Time - 50 min (10 min preparation)

Serves - 8-10 balls

250 g chestnut cooked peeled (you will get about 150-180 g chestnut after cooked and peeled)
3 tbsp almond butter
1 tbsp date puree or maple syrup
1/2 tsp salt
3 tbsp gluten-free oat flour (or pea protein powder or freeze dried fruit powder such as strawberry)
Cacao, desiccated coconut or edible glitter to roll

Using a small, sharp knife, cut a cross into the skin of each chestnut.
Put in a deep pot, cover with cold water and boil them until skins open and the insides are soft, about 30 minutes. Then peel them.

Put peeled chestnuts in a food processor, process until you get fine fresh chestnut flour.

Then add the almond butter, date puree, salt and oat flour (or protein powder or fruit powder). Process until everything combined well and smooth.

Transfer mixture in a bowl. Place in the freezer for 10-12 minutes. Once done, remove from the freezer, using a small icecream or cookie scopper, scoop out small balls. Roll with your hands into desiccated coconut, cacao or edible glitter.

Always store in the fridge. Once served, eat immediately.

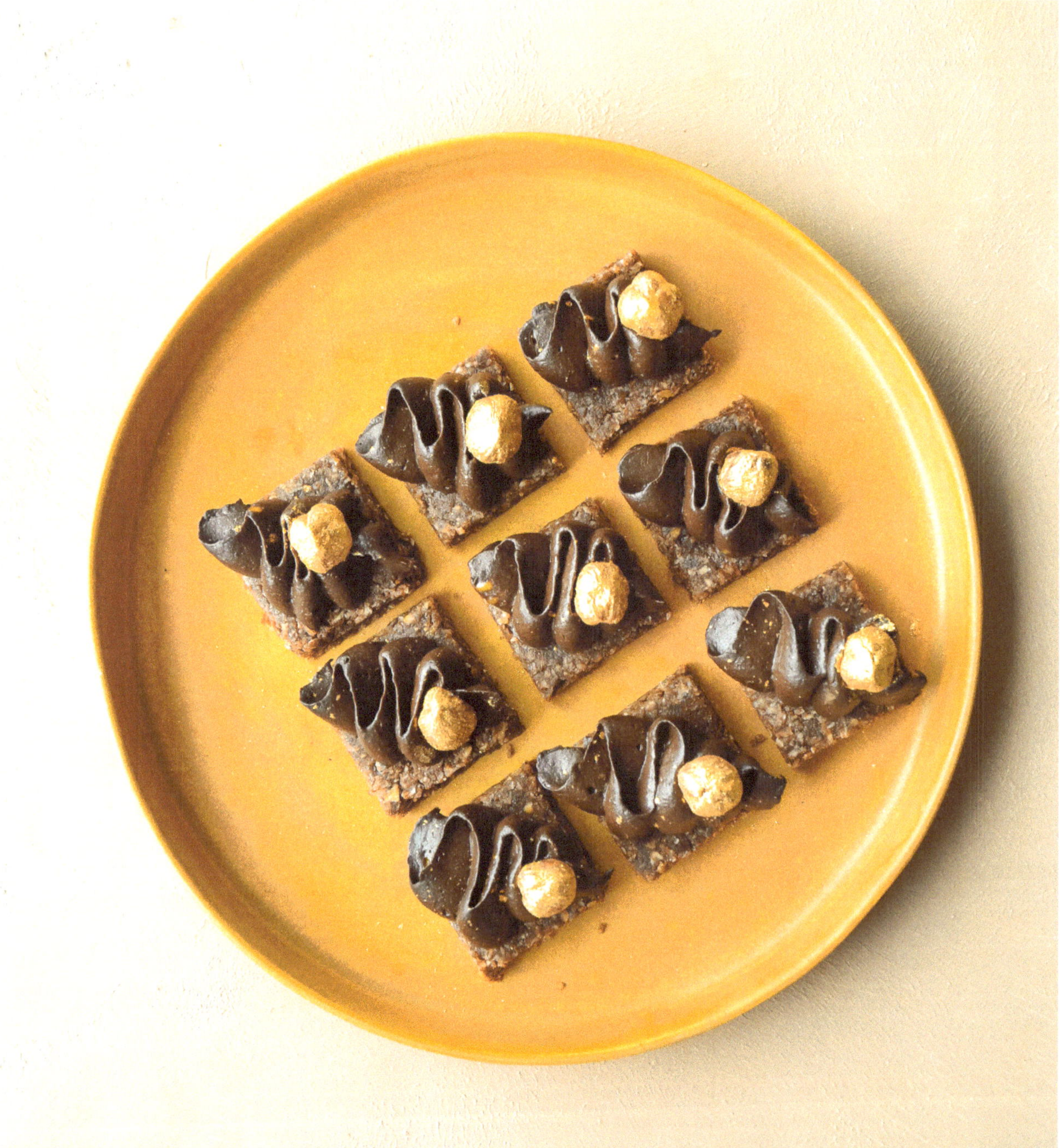

RAW BLONDIES WITH CHOCOLATE FROSTING

Time - 30 minutes
Serves - 18 squares

90 g gluten-free rolled oats
140 g smooth hazelnut butter
1/4 tsp pink himalayan salt
1 tsp vanilla bean powder
1 tsp raw cacao
3-4 tbsp hazelnut milk
1/2 cup hazelnuts to decorate

Avocado Frosting
1 perfectly ripe avocado
1 tbsp raw cacao powder
30 g melted raw chocolate
4 tbsp date puree or 2 tbsp maple
A pinch salt
1/4 vanilla bean powder
1 drop orange essential oil

Place rolled oats, salt, vanilla and cacao in the food processor, blend to combine.

Then add the hazelnut butter and milk. Process until you get a dough.

Transfer mixture in a 20x20 cm baking tin lined parchment paper. Press down the dough. Using a spatula, flatten out. Set in the refrigerator, while you are making the frosting.

To make avocado frosting, halve and pit the avocados, then scoop them into a food processor fitted with a steel blade or high-powered blender.

Add the raw cacao powder, orange essential oil, maple, melted chocolate, vanilla extract, and salt. Blend until very smooth and creamy, stopping to scrape down the bowl as needed.

Taste and add a few teaspoons of maple if additional sweetness is desired.

Transfer frosting in a pipping bag with wilton petal piping tip no 125, let it cool in the refrigerator for about 10 minutes.

Meanwhile, cut your brownies in small squares. Then decorate your brownies with the frosting. Top with hazelnuts.

TIPS

If you don't have piping tip, just by using a spatula, spread the frosting over the blondies.

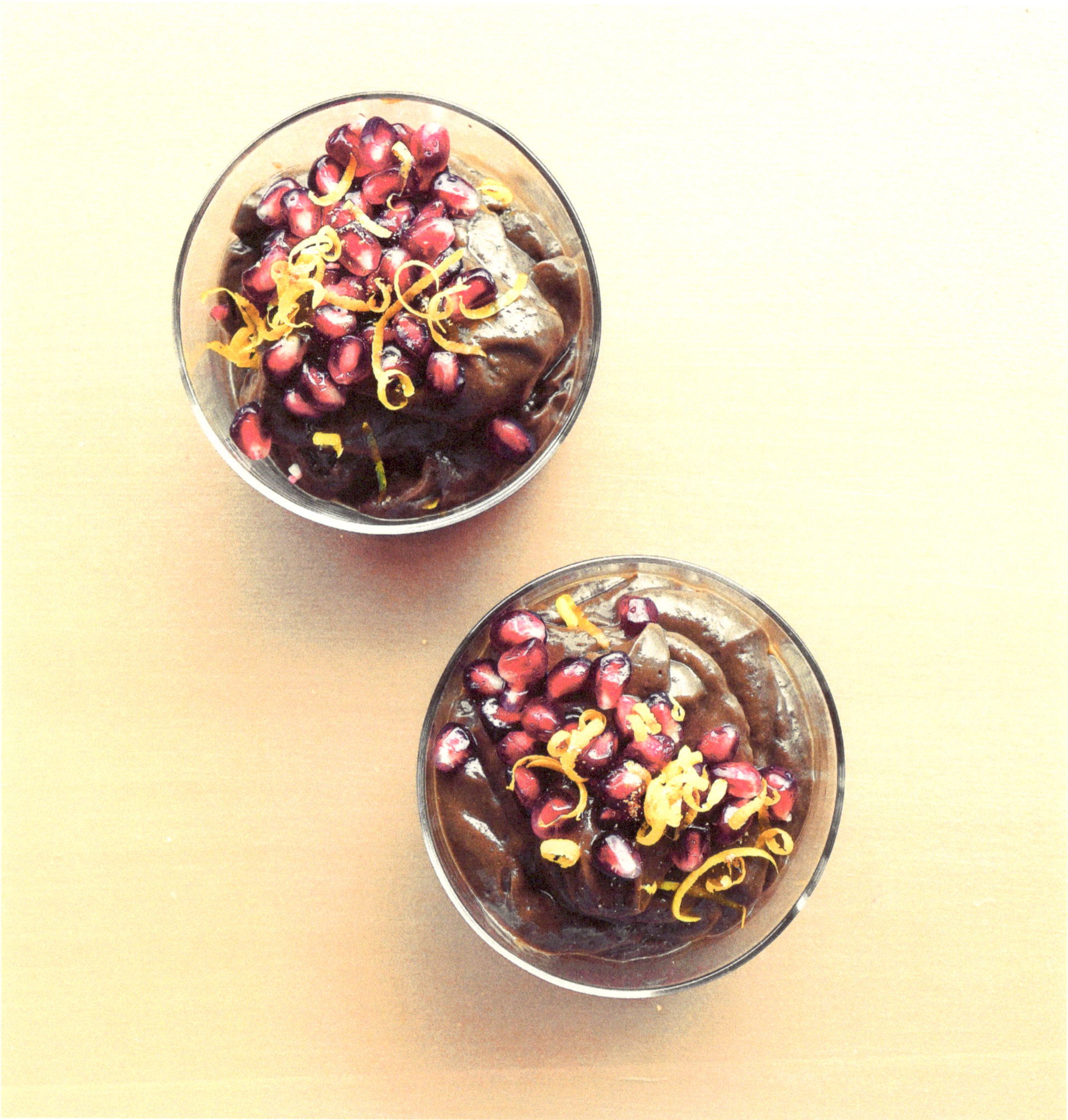

NO BAKE AVOCADO CHOCOLATE PUDDING

Beyond being delightfully healthful, this pudding also requires no cooking. Your prep tool will be a food processor or blender, and once chilled, the mousse will be everything you expect from the regular version of the decadent dessert; fluffy, deep in chocolate flavor, and high enough in fat to provide the same mouth feel you expect from a chocolate pudding.

Time - 10 minutes
Serves - 3-4 person

110 g ripe avocados (1 ripe avocado, measured after deseeded)
160 g ripe bananas (1.5-2 small bananas measured after peeled)
1/2 cup unsweetened almond milk (4 pieces almond + 1/2 cup water blended together)
1/4 cup raw cacao powder
6 fresh dates pitted and chopped + 1 tbsp maple if needed
1 tsp orange or lemon zest plus more for garnish
1/2 cup pomegranate seeds to serve
A pinch of salt
1/4 tsp cinnamon powder

In a blender or food processor combine avocados, bananas and plant milk. Blend until smooth, adding more milk if needed to reach desired consistency.

Add the rest of the ingredients and blend until smooth.

Spoon into jars or serving dishes. Cover and chill at least 4 hours.

To serve, top with pomegranate seeds. If desired, garnish with additional orange zest.

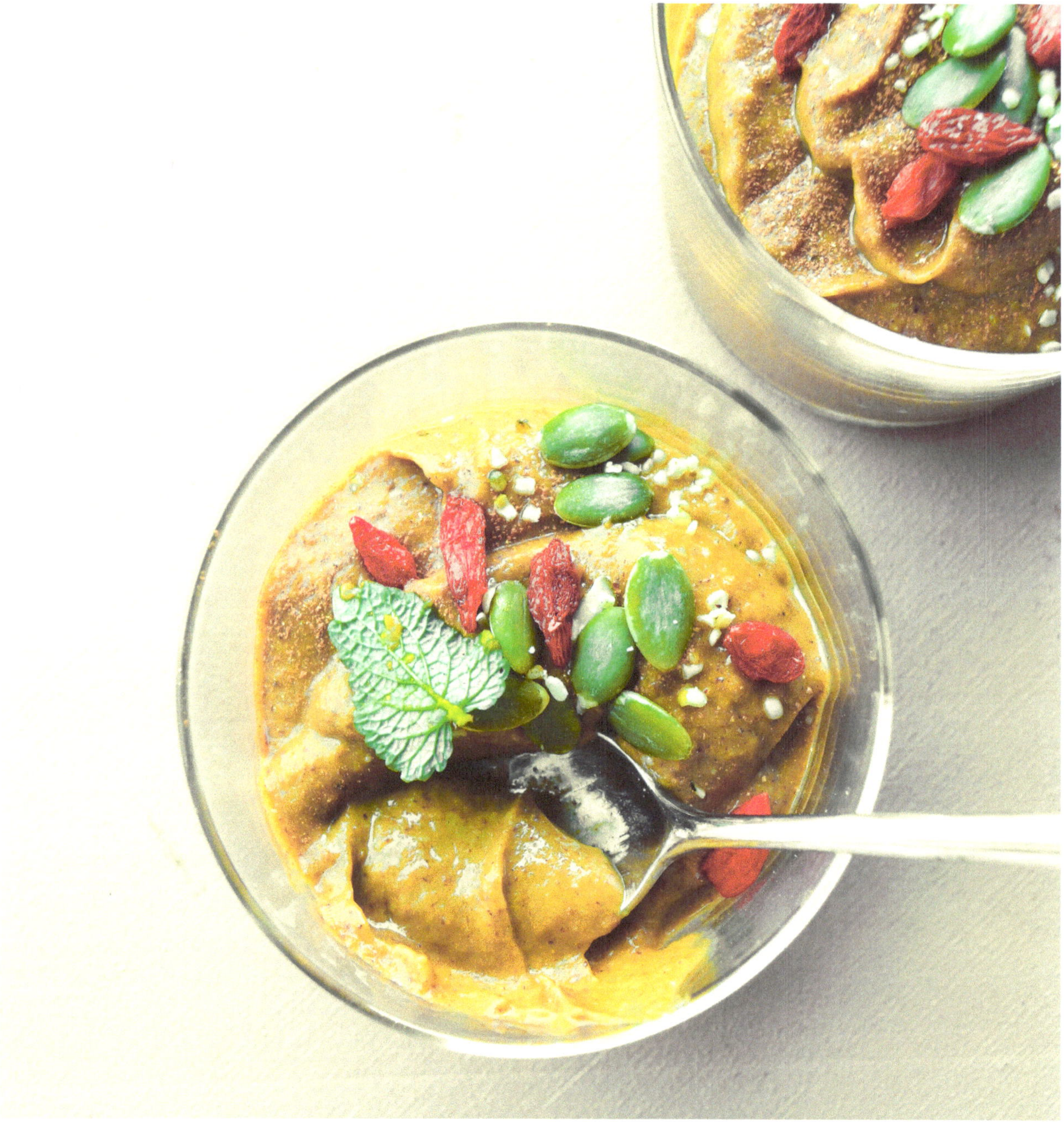

PUMPKIN PIE PUDDING

This semi-raw pumpkin pie pudding is healthy and delicious, like pumpkin pie without the crust! So fluffy, easy to make. The only cooked ingredient is pumpkin here. You can prepare it beforehand and make within 3 days.

Time - 10 minutes
Serves - 4 person

2 just-ripe bananas (180 g)
1/2 ripe avocado (100 g) pitted and peeled
3/4 cup pumpkin (180 g) puree (roast your own pumpkin and make the purée yourself)
1/4 cup almond butter
3-4 tbsp maple syrup (depending on how sweet you prefer)
50 g pitted soft sukkari dates (measured after seeds removed)
2 tsp pumpkin pie spice
1 tsp raw cacao
1/4 tsp pink himalayan salt
Crushed nuts to top of your choice (pumpkin seeds, walnuts, pecans and brazil nuts are the best options with this pudding)

Add the bananas, avocado, pumpkin puree, almond butter, maple syrup, pumpkin pie spice, vanilla, and sea salt to a food processor. Process for 2 minutes or until smooth and creamy, stopping to scrape down the sides as needed.

Divide between four serving glasses. You can enjoy the pudding as is; however, it thickens as it chills, so I recommend refrigerating it for at least 2 hours before serving.

Add desired toppings and serve.

It can be stored in an airtight container in the fridge up to 3-4 days.

TIPS

If you have time, try making this pudding on the day before you plan to serve it. Giving it additional time to set will improve the flavour of the spices and the consistency of the pudding.

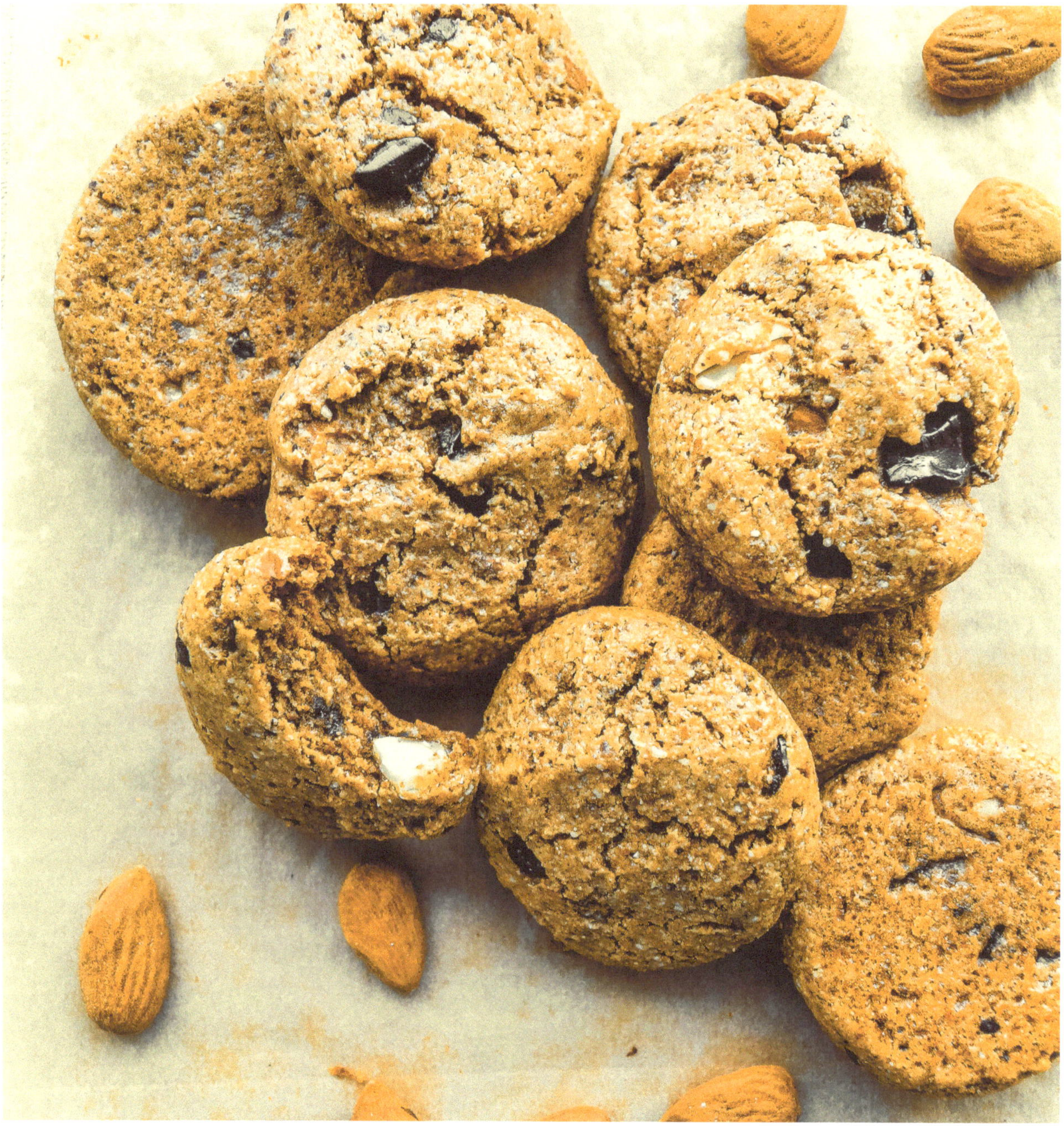

ALMOND BUCKWHEAT COOKIES

Time - 10 min prep + 20 min baking
Serves - makes 12 cookies

1/2 cup almond flour
1/2 cup sprouted buckwheat flour
4 tbsp almond butter
1/3 cup date paste
1 tbsp maple syrup
1 flax egg (1 tbsp ground flaxseeds mixed with 3 tbsp water)
1/2 tsp baking soda
1/2 tsp vanilla bean powder
A pinch of salt
1/4 cup chopped almonds
1/4 cup chopped vegan chocolate or raisins of your choice

Preheat oven to 175° C.

Using a coffee grinder, grind 1 tbsp flaxseed, transfer to a small bowl, add 3 tbsp water and let it sit for 3-4 minutes.

In a mixing bowl, add the almond flour, buckwheat flour, salt, vanilla bean powder and baking soda, whisk well.

Then add the almond butter, date paste, maple syrup and flaxseed mixture. Stir well until well combined.

Add the chopped almonds, chocolate or raisins, knead with your hands.

Make small balls from the dough. Press down to shape.

Transfer to a baking tray lined parchment paper.

Bake at 175° C for 20 minutes or until the top is golden brown. Remove from the oven and let cool.

Storage: They keep for up to 3 days at room temperature.

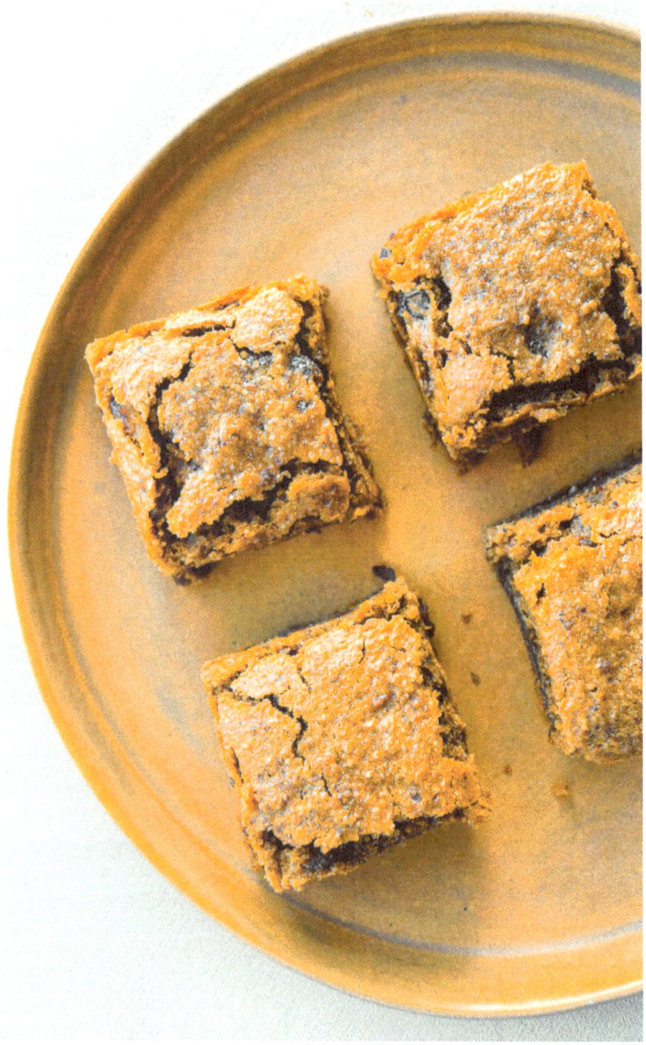

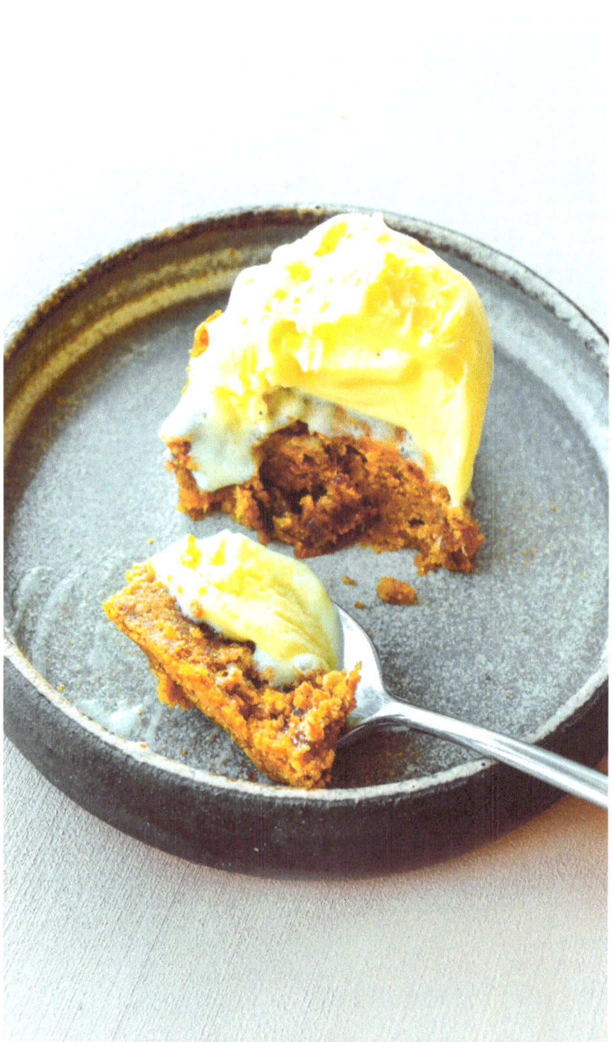

PUMPKIN BLONDIES

These blondies taste so good when you pair with a tangy ice cream. Try no ice cream machine needed recipe below or serve with your favorite plant-based ice cream.

Time - 15 min prep + 35 min baking
Serves - 6 person

55 g almond butter
110 g medjool dates purée (110g dates + 4 tbsp water blended)
60 g pumpkin purée
1 tbsp ground flaxseed + 3 tbsp water blended
3 tbsp maple syrup
100 g almond flour
100 g gluten-free oat flour
50 g tapioca flour or cassava
1 tsp baking powder
1/2 tsp salt
1/2 cup dried raisins soaked
1 tsp cinnamon
1/4 tsp cardamom
A pinch of nutmeg

Lemon Ice Cream
200 ml coconut butter (or almond butter)
200 ml coconut milk (or almond milk)
1/2 cup medjool dates pitted
3 tbsp maple syrup
1 tsp turmeric powder
1-2 drops lemon essential oil
1 tbsp lemon zest
A pinch salt

Preheat oven to 175° C.

In a large mixing bowl, mix the date purée, flax mixture, almond butter, maple syrup and pumpkin purée together.

In a separate bowl, whisk together almond flour, oat flour, tapioca, baking powder, salt, cinnamon, cardamom and nutmeg. Fold dry ingredients into wet. Mix well. Lastly add the raisins and stir well.
Refrigerate dough for 30 minutes.
Transfer dough into a baking tin lined parchment paper. The dough will be sticky, and that's okay. Use a spatula to spread the dough.
Bake for 25 minutes, until the cake is just set. Let cool on pan for 5 minutes, then move to a wire rack to finish cooling. Serve with lemon flavoured ice cream or your favorite one.

To make lemon ice cream, puree ingredients in a high speed blender until smooth.
Pour into a metal bowl and chill in the freezer, whipping with a silicone spatula every 15 minutes until it reaches desired consistency. Serve with your cake.

Storage: The cake will keep well in a closed container for up to 5 days.

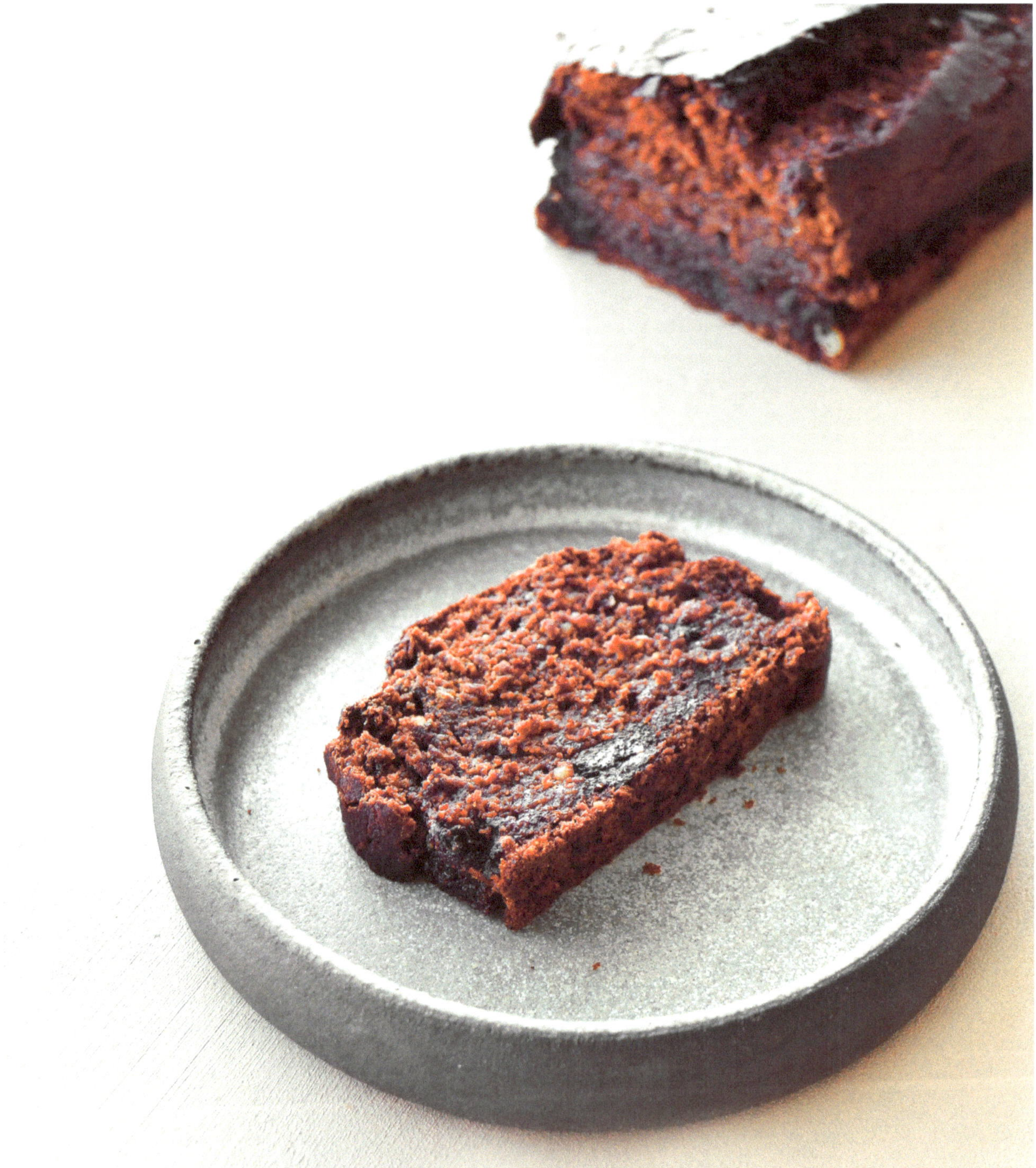

ZUCCHINI CHOCOLATE BREAD

Time - 1 hour
Serves - 8 -9 slices

2 tbsp flaxseed + 6 tbsp water
1 medium red apple + 1/4 cup water
120 ml maple syrup
1/4 cup hazelnut butter
1 tsp baking soda
1/4 tsp salt
1 cup grated zucchini
1/2 cup raw cacao powder or carob
90 g cassava or tapioca flour
35 g hazelnut flour
35 g gluten-free oat flour
40 g gluten-free vegan chocolate chopped or raspberry jam without sugar

Preheat your oven to 190° C.
Line a 9×5-inch loaf pan with parchment paper.
Grind your flaxseed in a coffee grinder. Place the flax meal in a mixing bowl, add the water. Let it rest for 5 minutes.

Meanwhile core the apple and discard. Cut the apple into small pieces, place in a high speed blender, add the water. Blend until you get smooth puree. Once done, transfer to your mixing bowl.
Next add the hazelnut butter and whisk to combine. Add grated zucchini and stir to combine.

Add the hazelnut flour, oat flour and cassava, whisk until just combined. The batter should be scoopable and thick. Lastly add the chopped chocolate and stir well.

Bake 1 hour or until a toothpick comes out clean.
Let it cool at least 15-20 minutes before cutting. It is best when refrigerated for 2-3 hours and then sliced. Texture is wonderful and easy to cut when cooled completely.

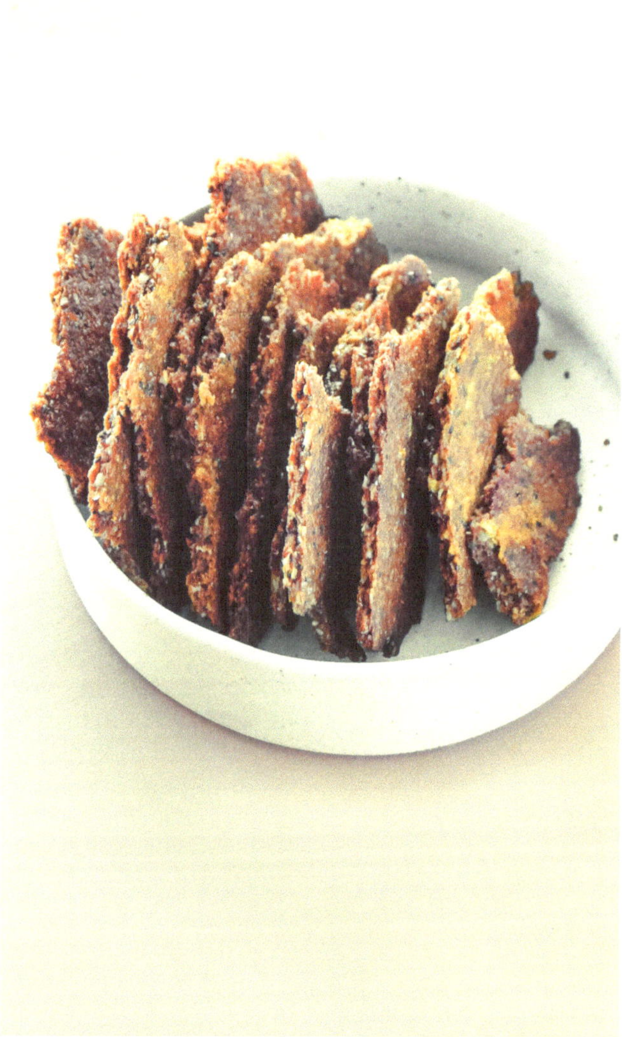

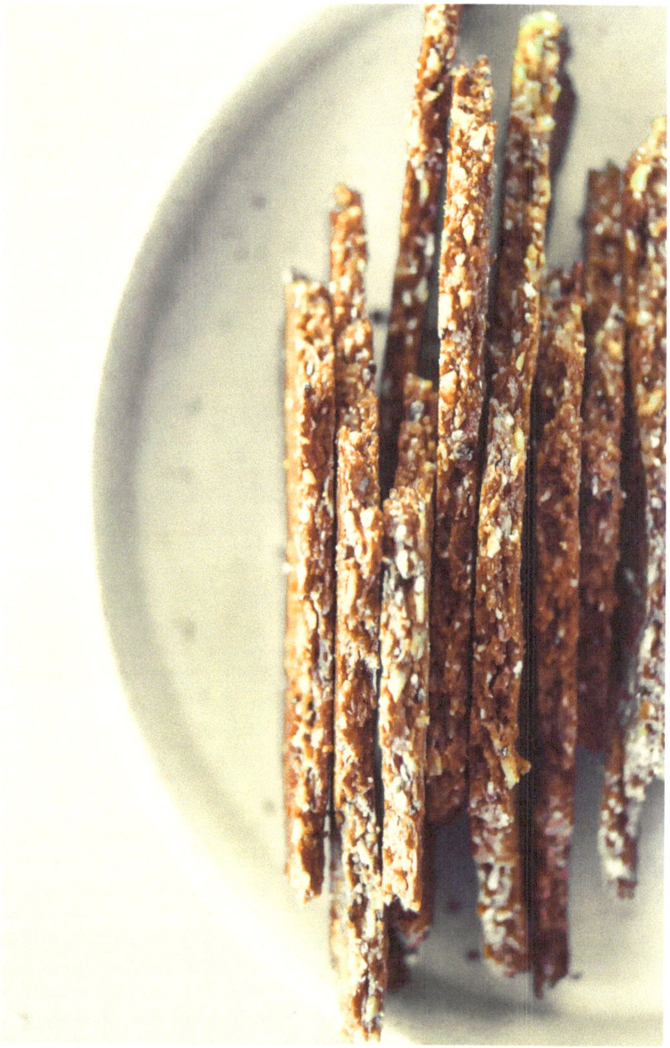

OAT HAZELNUT THINS

Have you ever wondered what happens when you bake bliss balls? I did. The result is here, delicious thin crispy snacks! This multi-functional recipe can also be made by forming dough balls without cooking process. Both are so delicious and easy to make!

Time - 35 min
Serves - 4-6

80 g gluten-free rolled oats
10 g chia seeds
135 g hazelnut butter
1-2 tbsp plant milk (or water)
3 tbsp maple
A pinch salt

Preheat oven to 180° C.

Place the oats, chia seeds and salt in the food processor, blitz until slightly flour.

Add the hazelnut butter, maple and plant milk. Process until everything combined well. You should get a sticky dough.

Using two parchment paper and a rolling pin, roll the dough between parchment, as thin as possible.

Bake in the oven for 13-15 minutes. Let it cool at least 15 minutes before breaking in pieces.

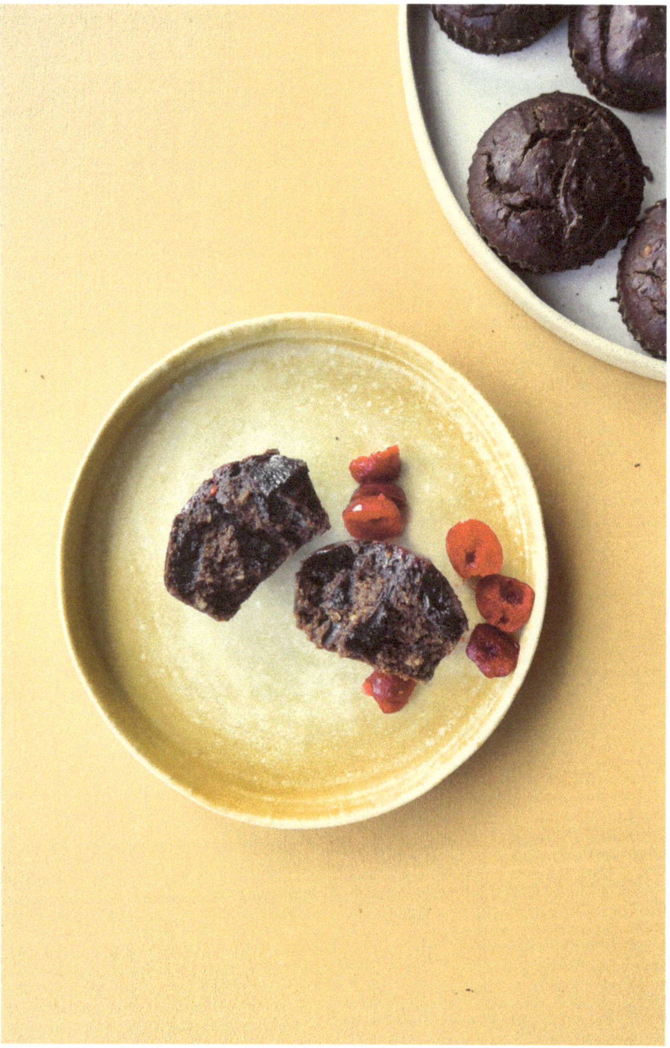

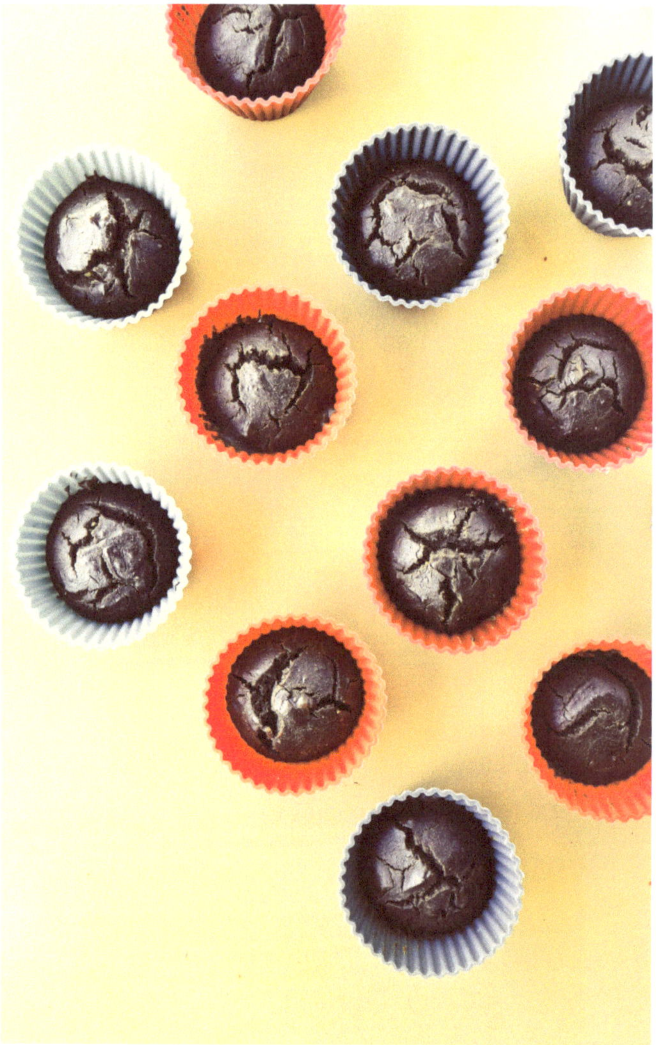

TEFF CHOCOLATE MUFFINS

Made with the nutrient-dense whole grain, teff. Soft and moist, with cherries and lemon.

Time - 35 min
Serves - 4-6

1 ground flaxseed + 3 tbsp water (you can sub the flax with chia seeds, if so you don't need to grind them)
175 ml almond milk
110 ml maple syrup (or grape molasses)
1/3 cup almond butter
1 tsp vanilla bean powder
1 tsp apple cider vinegar
1 cup (150 g) teff flour
1/4 cup (50 g) tapioca (or cassava)
1/4 cup (25 g) cacao powder
1/2 tsp baking soda
1/4 tsp salt
50 g gluten-free vegan chocolate chopped

Cherry Coulis
1 cup fresh or defrosted cherries
1 tbsp maple syrup (or grape molasses)
1 tbsp chia seeds
1 tbsp lemon juice

Preheat oven to 180° C.

Put the ground flax with the water in a bowl, mix and let stand for 5-10 minutes.

Mix all the wet ingredients; almond milk, maple, almond butter, apple cider vinegar and add the flax mixture to them.
In another bowl, mix the dry ingredients; teff flour, tapioca, cacao, baking soda, salt, vanilla bean powder.

Pour the wet batter to dry, add the chopped chocolate and stir to combine. Then fill the muffin tins to three-quarters the height. Transfer as quickly as possible to the hot oven.
After 25 minutes check if a toothpick comes out clean, if not give a few more minutes, then take out, and wait for them to cool completely before.

Place all cherry coulis in a mixing bowl, mix well and let it sit for 15 minutes until thicken but still liquid enough to pour. Using a piping bag with round tip or syringe, push the cherry coulis into muffins. You can also serve them with fresh cherries. Do not skip the cherries. This tangy flavour adds another dimension to muffins.
They can be stored in the refrigerator in an airtight container up to 4-5 days.

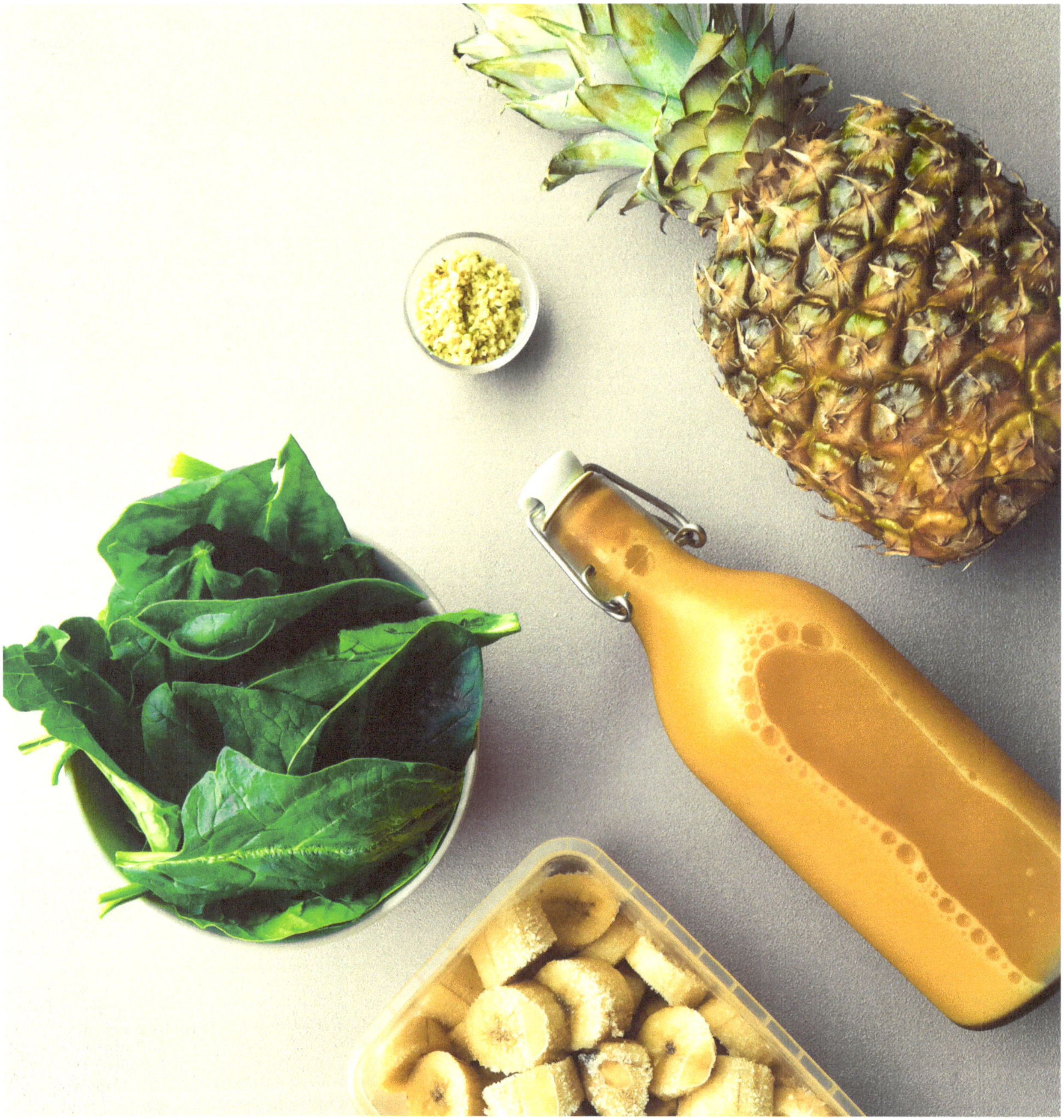

THE WISE SMOOTHIE

If you're looking for the new ways of including more greens in your meals but can't eat a lot in a salad form, this smoothie is a smart savior. I call this "wise smoothie" because this combo tastes super good and works with any kind of greens such as celery, kale, collard greens, swiss chard, spinach...

Time - 10 minutes
Serves - 4 person

400 g frozen bananas
1 ripe pineapple
A handful of fresh spinach (or tuscan kale, celery, collard, chard)
500 ml fresh orange juice with 1 tbsp freshly grated or juiced ginger
2-3 tbsp hemp hearts

Peel and cut your pineapple into small pieces.

Wash and drain your kale leaves.

Juice fresh orange juice about 400-500 ml depending on the liquid consistency you like.

Peel and grate your ginger.

Place all the ingredients in a high speed blender. Blend until smooth.
Divide between the glasses, enjoy!

MINI CINNAMON RAISIN CAKE WITH PUMPKIN FROSTING

Time - 15 min prep + 30 min baking

Serves - 4-5 slices

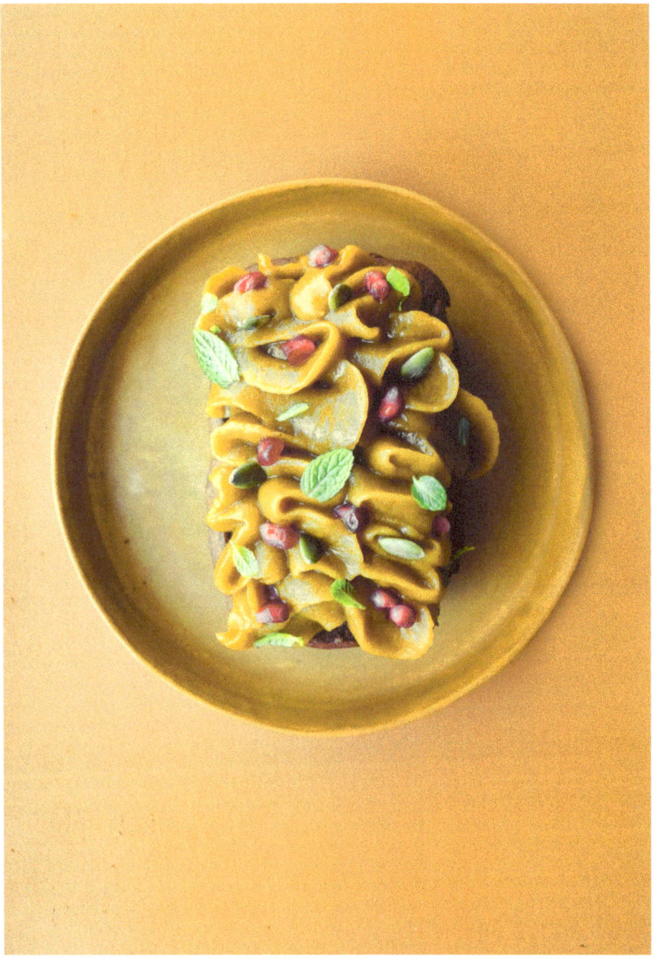

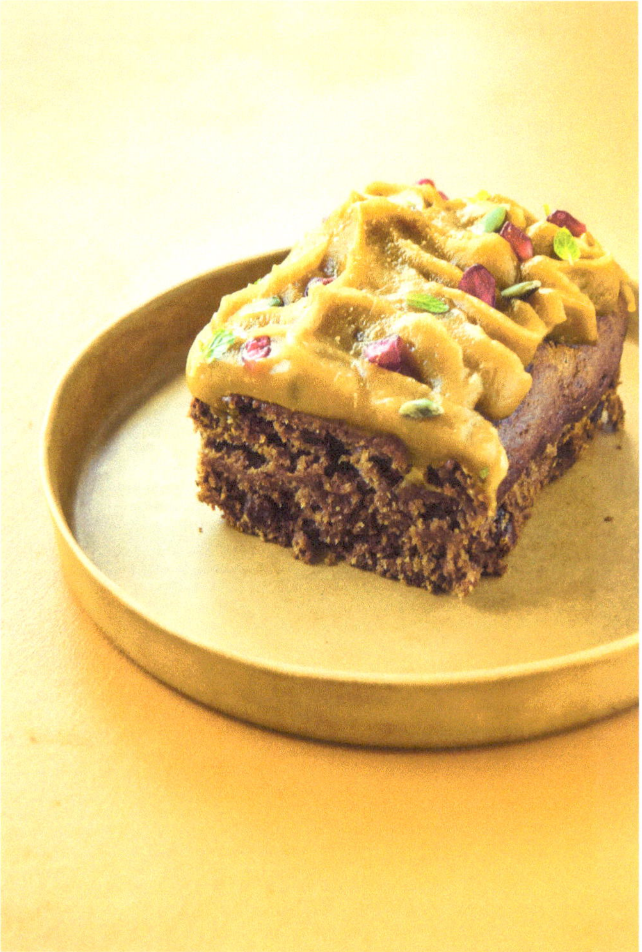

Less is more. I have created this recipe made of simple, healthy and complementing ingredients which allow individual flavors to stand out. I love the subtle sweetness of the dates with the tangy orange zest. Combined with nutty almond butter adds protein as well as an earthy flavour. Topped with silky smooth pumpkin cream.

70 g gluten-free oat flour
60 g grape molasses
75 g mashed bananas
35 g almond butter
30 g dried raisins
1 tsp apple cider vinegar
1 g cinnamon
2 tbsp orange zest
A pinch salt
1 tsp baking soda
50 g almond milk
1/4 cup pomegranates to garnish

Pumpkin Frosting
70 g cooked pumpkins
80 g fresh sukkari dates
60 g almond milk
1 tbsp grape molasses
2 tbsp espresso (or plant milk)
A pinch salt
1/4 tsp cinnamon powder

Place the bananas in a mixing bowl, mash using a fork. Then add the almond butter, apple cider vinegar and grape molasses. Stir to combine together well.
Add the cinnamon, orange zest, baking soda, salt and almond milk. Mix well until everything combined well.
Lastly add the oat flour and mix together.
Line a mini cake tin with parchment paper. I used 15x10 cm rectangle tin. Pour the cake batter in the tin.

Bake at 190° C for 25-30 minutes or until a knife or toothpick inserted in the center comes out clean, then remove from the oven. Allow the tin to cool for about 10 minutes.
Flip the tin over a plate and pop out the cake. Be careful because they are very light and fluffy. Then transfer them to a wire rack to cool.

Meanwhile, start making pumpkin frosting. Cook the pumpkins until tender fork. In a small food blender (I used blendtec twister jar), add all the pumpkin frosting ingredients. Blend until silky smooth. Close the lid of the jar. Store in the fridge to set a bit until the desired consistency is reached.
Once cake is done, remove from the tin. Using a piping bag with wilton 125 tip, decorate your cake. If you don't have piping bag or tip, just spread the frosting over the cake. Garnish with pomegranates or pepitas if desired.
Storage: Although it is better the day of or day after baking, it can be stored in the fridge for up to 3-4 days.

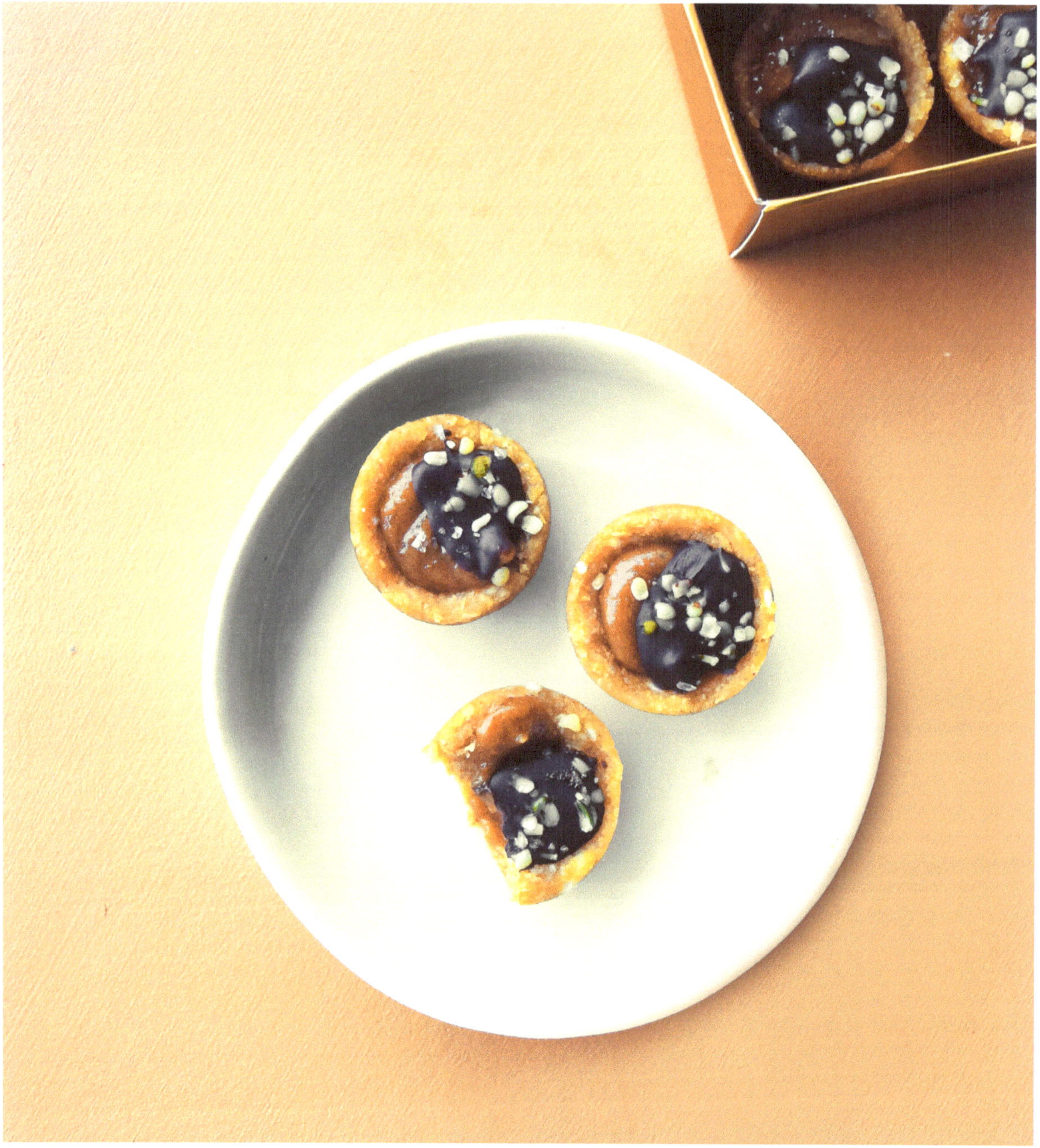

RAW TOFFEE CUPS

Time - 1 hour
Serves - 3 cm 20 pieces (I used Pralinform halvklot mold from Pufz.se)

Crust
70 g sprouted rolled oats
50 g activated dehydrated almonds
15 g psyllium husk powder
15 g desiccated coconut
15 g almond butter
40 g maple syrup
60 ml plant milk or water
1/4 tsp pink himalayan salt

Caramel
85 g soft medjool dates (weight after seeds removed), soaked
30 g dried raisins, soaked
50 g almond butter
50 g maple
1 tsp cinnamon powder
1/4 tsp salt

Chocolate
60 g melted raw chocolate
Hemp hearts to decorate

To make crust, place the oats, almonds in a high speed blender, process until you get powder. Then transfer mixture to a food processor, add the psyllium husk, desiccated coconut and salt, process until everything combined well. Add the almond butter, maple syrup and plant milk. Continue to mix until you get a dough-form. If it is too wet, add more desiccated coconut, if it is too dry, add extra plant milk, one tablespoon at a time.
Once done, take a teaspoon from the dough and fill the cavities of the mold. Use a teaspoon for each cavity. Press down with your hands and leave the middle of the cavities empty to fill with the caramel sauce.

Soak your raisins and dates in warm water for 20 minutes then strain and dry. Transfer to a high speed blender (I used Blendtec with twister jar). Add the rest of the ingredients. Blend until everything combined well and you get a silky smooth caramel consistency.
Transfer mixture in a piping bag, alternatively you can use a teaspoon to fill the middle of the cavities.
Repeat the process for the rest.

Using a bain marie method, melt the raw chocolate. Add 1/2 to 1 tsp chocolate (cover all or half of the top with chocolate). Sprinkle some hemp hearts over the chocolate.

Freeze for 1 hour or keep in the refrigerator for 2-3 hours or until completely cooled. Then remove from the mold.

OAT WALNUT CRUMBLE WITH BERRIES

Time - 30 min prep + 4 hrs setting

Serves - 15 cm round cake

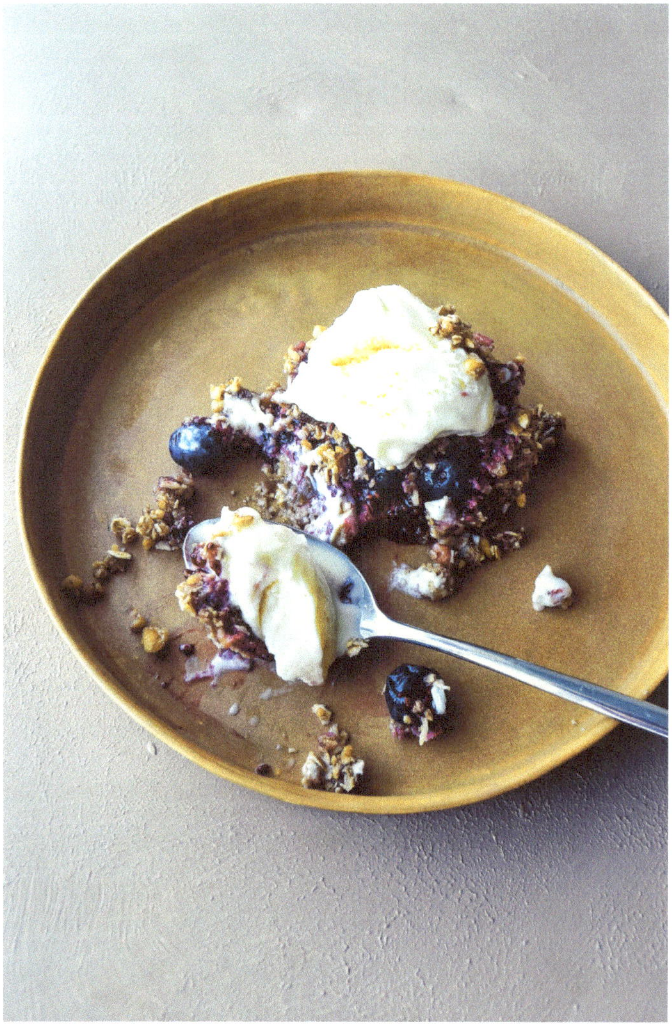

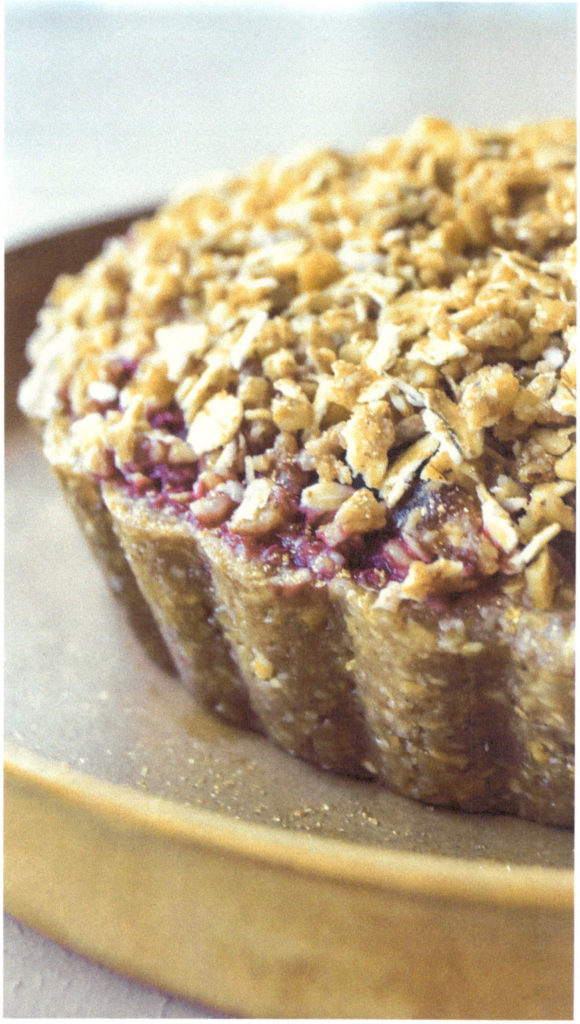

Crust

130 g gluten-free rolled oats
65 g walnut flour
65 g desiccated coconut
1 tbsp coconut flour
1 tbsp water
1 tbsp coconut butter (or almond butter)
5 tbsp date paste
1/2 tsp vanilla bean powder
1 tsp cinnamon powder
1/2 tsp ginger powder
1/4 tsp cardamom
A pinch nutmeg
A pinch of pink himalayan salt

Crumble on top

65 g gluten-free rolled oats
130 g walnuts
1 tbsp coconut flour
2 tbsp date paste
2 medjool dates finely pitted
1 tbsp desiccated coconut
1 tbsp coconut butter (or almond butter)
1/2 tsp cinnamon powder
1/4 tsp ginger powder
1/4 tsp cardamom
A pinch nutmeg
A pinch licorice salt (or pink himalayan)

Coconut Ice Cream to Serve

200 g fair-trade young coconut meat (from the 2 young coconuts)
130 g plant milk
50 g sukkari or medjool date paste
2-3 tbsp lemon juice
1 tbsp coconut butter (or almond butter)

Berry Jam

200 mixed forest berries of your choice (blackberry, blueberry, raspberry, lingonberry etc.)
65 g dried raisins soaked
2 tbsp chia seeds
1 tbsp maple syrup
1 tbsp psyllium husk powder
1 tsp orange zest
1 tbsp grated fresh ginger

Instructions

Place all the ingredients for the cake crust ingredients in a food processor and process until they combine into a dough. Once done, remove from the food processor and knead a little with your hands. Place a parchment paper in a 15 cm cake or pie tin and press the dough evenly into the tin. Make a nice about 1 – 1.5 cm edge along the shape. Set in the freezer for 10-15 minutes meanwhile start making the jam.

To make jam, place berries and raisins in a bowl, add the rest of the ingredients for the filling berry jam. Mix well and let it sit while you are making the top crumble. To make top crumble, roughly mix all ingredients except oats in the food processor. Add oatmeal and pulse shredded 1-2 times. Remove from the food processor. Sprinkle the crumble on the berry jam layer. Let it sit for 1-2 hours in the fridge.

Place all the coconut ice cream ingredients into an ice cream maker or blender, blend until you get silky smooth mixture. Taste the mixture, if you need add more lemon juice and dates or 1-2 tbsp maple syrup. Then mix well and pour mixture in a rectangle mould. Freeze for 4-5 hours. Once done, using an ice cream scooper, scoop out and serve with your crumble cake.

INDEX

A

B

C

O

P

Q

R

S

"You leave a mark on every person that you meet. Leave people better than you found them."

- Newhappyco

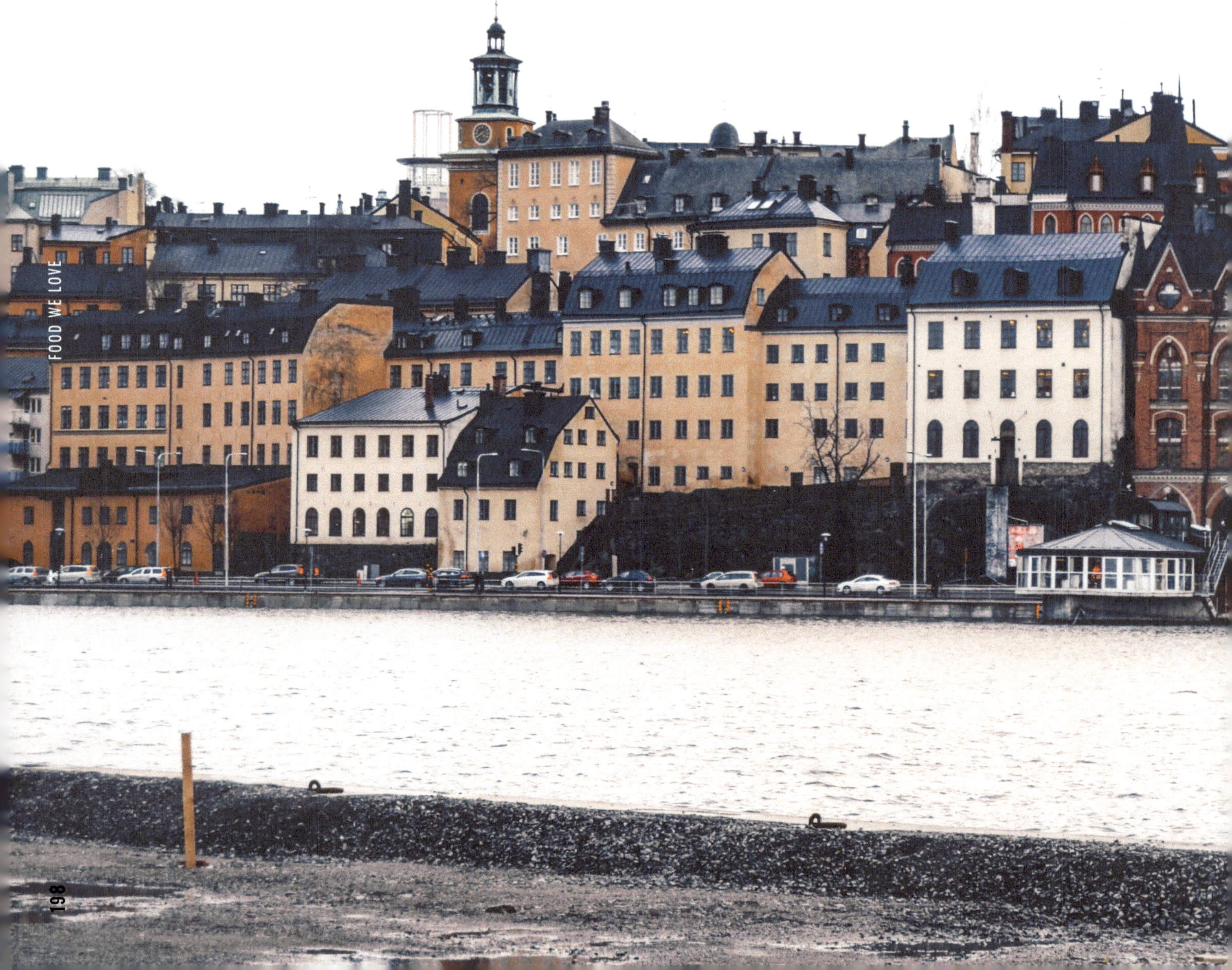

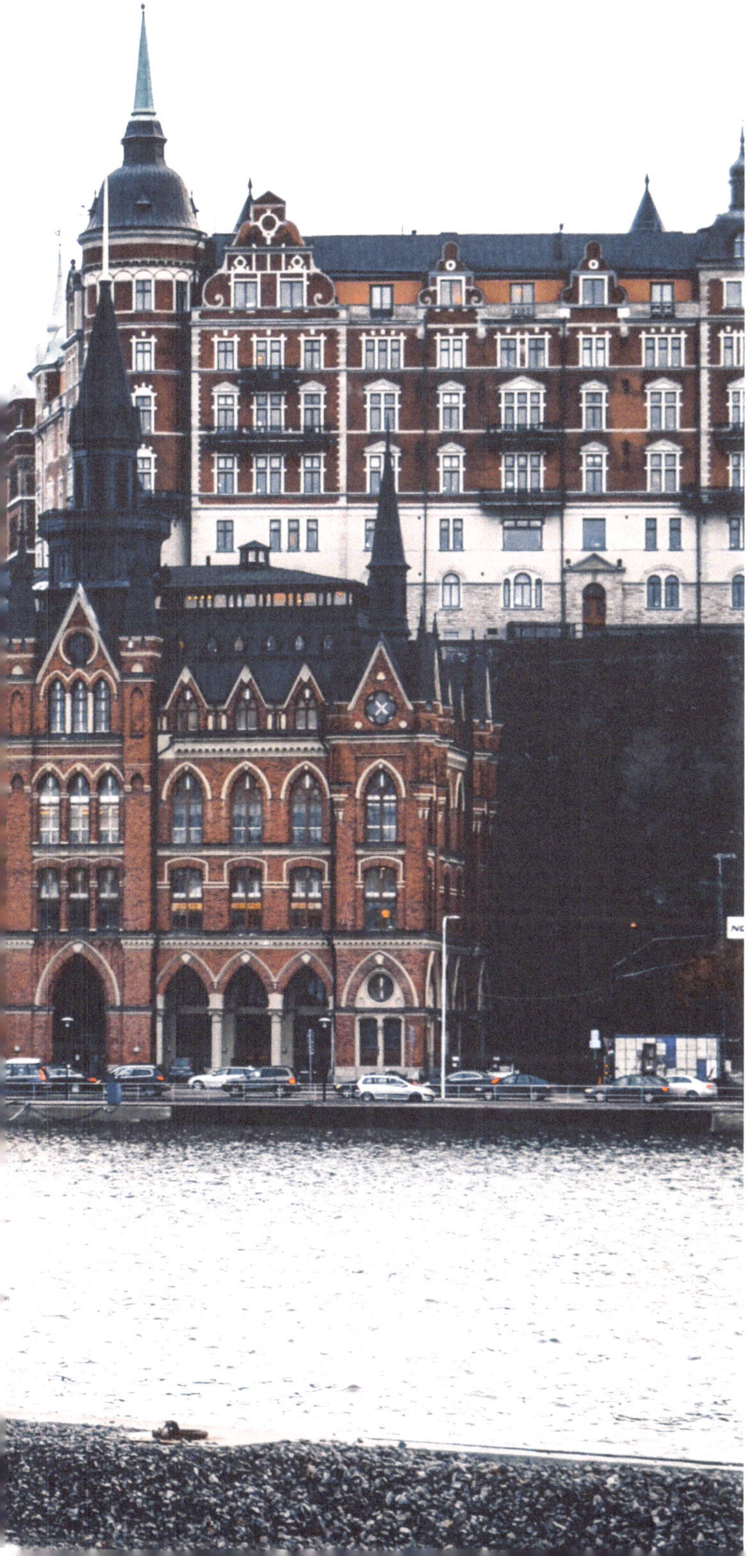

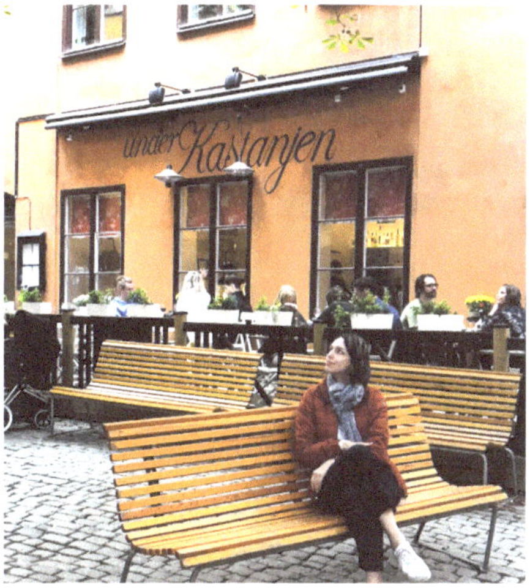

about the author

Nazlı Develi is a plant food designer, an inventive, aesthetically minded hands-on chef and artist with an eye for details and the founder of GREEN & AWAKE: Plant Food Design Studio.

She specialized in wholesome plant-based and raw cuisine, restaurant consultancy, recipe development, workshops, chef training and creative concepts, all rooted in food expression with nature as a core.

Obsessed with art, design, health, wellness and experimental flavours, she's strongly committed to spreading awareness about plant-based food as the most sustainable and necessary alternative for the planet.

Instagram: @gurmevegan I @greenandawake

Website: www.gurmevegan.com

www.greenandawake.com

www.ingramcontent.com/pod-product-compliance
Ingram Content Group UK Ltd.
Pitfield, Milton Keynes, MK11 3LW, UK
UKHW061539051026
15625UKWH00011B/533
9781736374290